Born Too Soon...

BUT NOT FOR A MIRACLE!

Cyndy Thomas

PO Box 133. Owasso, OK 74055

ISBN 978-0-9749084-6-5

Acknowledgment

My eternal gratitude to Steve and Fran Goodmon
and to Dave Giegerich,

without whom,
this book might never have been written,

and to our loving Father God,
without whom,
there wouldn't even be a story to tell.

Table of Contents

Preface

"HELP! ... SOMEONE HELP!" the delivery room nurse frantically yelled as she leaned toward the open doorway. While keeping one of her hands firmly braced on my leg to hold me on the delivery table, she stretched even closer to the door. ***"SOMEONE, PLEASE HELP!"***

I had never seen a nurse panic like that before. She and I had been left alone in the delivery room for only a few seconds, but it was clear to her that time had run out. My baby was going to be born, and it was happening RIGHT NOW!

Although this professionally skilled woman had assisted in countless deliveries over the years, this particular birth was causing her tremendous anxiety, because it was not a deli-very that could be managed single-handedly. My baby was making its grand entrance three months too soon, and this nurse knew it was a life or death situation.

Within seconds, in response to her cries, it seemed like hundreds of people came rushing through the open door, although it was actually more like eight or nine. Included in that group was a special team of five doctors and nurses from the intensive care nursery down the hall. They had all been hurriedly summoned to my bedside to receive the precious handoff at the moment of birth. The gynecologist and a few delivery room nurses made up the rest of the squad, and we were now in the final moments just before delivery. The team was in place with only seconds to spare.

How had I ended up in the middle of this frenzy that resembled a swarming beehive; and what was causing my baby to be born so early? Was there no way to prevent this premature birth? What in the world had gone wrong?

The sobering answers to these questions may astound you; and after hearing the details, you will understand why I say,

"My baby was born too soon ...
but not too soon for a miracle!"

Chapter 1

Surprises

The story of this miracle begins in early January of 1981. I had just received the glorious news from my gynecologist that a bundle of joy was on the way, and I was ecstatic! For several months, I had obediently followed the doctor's order to daily chart my morning temperature to determine if my reproductive organs were properly functioning. Now, I was being graced with the wonderful announcement that I would be having a baby!

Finally, after all the many months of effort, I could relax. Or could I? No one knew that some unexpected surprises were coming along with this bundle of joy.

Before I go any further with the story, though, some background information should be interjected here. A few months before I received the doctor's good news that I was expecting a baby, I had been involved in a minor car accident and had required some physical therapy for an injury to my lower back. The therapy included X-rays initially, then weekly heat and ultrasound treatments over the next several weeks.

I was given a medical form to complete at my first therapy session. Among the many questions on the form, one asked, *"Are you pregnant?"* My answer was, *"No."* I was not pregnant at the time of the wreck nor when my therapy began.

At some point after that, though, I did become pregnant while still undergoing those treatments. In hindsight, it now appears that the therapy treatments I received could have actually been the catalyst for the serious complications I later developed during my pregnancy.

The first clue that something was amiss showed up shortly after my initial visit to the gynecologist in January where I received confirmation that I was pregnant. A few weeks after that visit, amidst my joy and celebration, an alarming symptom appeared. I suddenly began to bleed as though I wasn't even pregnant.

Immediately, horrible thoughts stormed my mind, and fear rushed in like a flood. I had flashbacks to the time six years earlier when I had lost a baby three months into my first pregnancy. That miscarriage had started with an identical symptom, unexplained bleeding. I was not going to take any chances this time. So, I called my doctor's office to get emergency instructions.

Surprisingly, the nurse simply asked me a few questions over the phone, such as, *"Is the bleeding as heavy as your normal menstrual period would be?"* Since it wasn't, I said, *"No, not quite." "Well then,"* she calmly said, *"You should just go about your normal duties."* She didn't think the flow was enough to merit the doctor checking my condition nor for me to have a doctor's order for total bed rest.

That was it?! *"Just go about your normal duties."* Even though I was experiencing the same traumatic symptoms as my previous miscarriage, her advice to me was merely, *"Go about your normal duties."* I couldn't believe my ears. I have certainly learned a lot in the years since then, but at that time in my life, age 25, I wasn't one to openly question a doctor's or a nurse's instructions. I did wonder to myself, though, how she could possibly determine my exact condition by phone without some kind of examination? Wanting to be a good little patient, though, I felt compelled to oblige, so I blindly accepted her decision.

However, into the picture came my mother. Immediately upon hearing about the problem I was having, she quickly made plans for my brood to temporarily take up residence with her. She informed me that bed rest was precisely what I needed, in spite of the nurse's advice. Furthermore, she suggested that her house was where I would get the best rest, and she invited my family there.

My mother lived about 12 miles away in the next town, and she had been alone since my father's death six years earlier. I gladly welcomed the help she offered. So, Mother became my "Nurse Nancy" and also attended to the needs of my husband and my four-year-old son, Jeremy. Time would prove in this situation that Mother did know best.

With total bed rest, the hemorrhaging stopped within a week. By then, it was time for my regular monthly visit to the doctor. At that visit, I was surprised when he asked me if there had been any problems since my last appointment a month ago. He had my chart in his hands, and his question made me wonder whether there was any mention of my emergency phone call earlier about the bleeding.

I proceeded to explain what had transpired during the previous two weeks. After hearing details of my problem, he decided to do an internal exam, which I thought was strange. It seemed to me that you wouldn't want to do anything to cause further bleeding. But once again, what did I know? I wasn't the professional. He was. I was only the patient.

After the exam, the doctor stood facing me. I will never forget the words he spoke to me at the end of my exam that day. He looked me straight in the face, never changing his facial expression, and declared in his monotone, *"Well, you could still lose your baby."*

I was stunned and devastated. With no compassion whatsoever in his voice, he didn't even preface the dark announcement by saying he was sorry to have to tell me such bad news. His words were blunt, cold, matter-of-fact, and seemed very easy for him to say.

After dropping that bombshell on me, and with no further explanation as to what was wrong with me, he left. The office visit was over. I was left alone in that small exam room with his devastating news and a horrible heaviness. His gloom-filled words hung over me like a dark cloud of painful hopelessness. Even now, I can remember staring at the printed blue wallpaper and feeling like my entire world was spinning out of control.

Somehow, I managed to get out of that paper gown and dress myself in spite of the nausea that was creeping into my stomach. I walked out of that office in a puzzled daze. After all, when I had called about the bleeding two weeks earlier, there seemed to be very little concern on their part. Remember, I was told to simply go about my normal duties. But now, I was being told the exact opposite - that I could easily lose this precious gift I was carrying.

Something was terribly wrong with this picture. In hindsight, I realize this should have been my first clue to "Run, don't walk, to the nearest exit" to find a new doctor. If I'd known then what I know now, I would've done exactly that.

A cycle of bleeding between each of my monthly appointments became a matter of routine. The bleeding happened once or twice every month just like clockwork. Each time it started, I followed the same procedure. I called the doctor's office and got the same response, *"Go about your normal duties."* But instead, I would listen to my heart, not that doctor. So, on a regular basis, my little flock and I would temporarily move into my mom's house, and I would retire to her back bedroom for bed rest.

During the many months of this bleeding disorder, my octor never scheduled an ultrasound exam for me. That simple medical procedure had become commonplace for pregnancies by this time. If this one simple test had been performed at any point during my pregnancy, it would have shown exactly what was causing the bleeding.

Instead, each month at my regular office visit, I was routinely given an internal exam and heard the same words from that doctor again and again. *"You could still lose your baby."* None of this made any sense to me, but at that stage of my young life, I was not comfortable questioning a doctor. So, I just suffered through all of it. Many times since then, though, I've wished that I had confronted this doctor's negligence. But, of course, hindsight is 20/20.

Chapter 2

Shock

In the midst of this chaos, something good was happening on another front. Early into this pregnancy, I found out I would soon be the proud owner of my first home! What an exciting, extraordinary time this was turning out to be.

Our trusty, two-bedroom mobile home had served its purpose, but it was time to move up. The new house was an older, remodeled one located in the same town as my mom. It had a fenced yard that would be perfect for Jeremy and the new baby. However, getting the new baby here safely was becoming a major task that overshadowed everything, even moving to the new house.

Just when I needed to be packing for the move, the bleeding started again, and I was forced to stay off my feet. That meant other people had to do the things that I should have been doing.

I have very vivid memories of my son, age four, sitting on the floor watching television while I was lying on the couch near him, trying to prevent further pregnancy complications. The packing and moving was going on all around us.

Toward the last of the move, when it was time to take the couch and the bed from the mobile home, my family and I once again took up residence temporarily at my mom's. This allowed me to stay off my feet until things became normal at the new house, although "normal" was not what it used to be. The move into our new house took place in

February. We had no way of knowing what would occur in just a few short months.

The doctor had set September 1 as the due date for my baby's birth. Given the monthly complications I was experiencing, that date seemed years away, because it took a huge amount of effort every day to sustain this pregnancy. In late May, the unthinkable happened.

During the early morning hours of Monday, May 25, I was sleeping soundly in bed in our new home. I was abruptly awakened around 1 AM as though someone had called my name or shaken me. After listening for a moment to determine the cause of my awakening, and finding none, I made one of my frequent nighttime trips to the bathroom located just a few steps from the bed.

As soon as I was seated in the bathroom, my world spun completely out of control. Suddenly, a huge clot of blood passed from my body, and a stream of blood began to flow. At that moment, I thought I had just given birth in my bathroom and was now bleeding to death.

I yelled for my husband who came running, bleary-eyed from a sound sleep. He grabbed a large bath towel and quickly escorted me the short distance back to bed. As I lay there, I wondered if I was in fact bleeding to death. My husband was hurriedly calling an ambulance and then my doctor. The doctor told him to have me transported to the large hospital where he practiced about 30 miles away.

When the paramedics arrived, they took my vitals and checked the towel to determine the amount of blood loss. They quickly loaded me into the ambulance, which was an older station wagon type, and we began the rush to the hospital. That was my first and only ambulance ride, and honestly, I wasn't sure which condition might kill me first, the blood loss or the terrible exhaust fumes I was breathing from the vehicle that had been sent to save my life!

My eyes were closed most of the time, and I don't recall the ambulance attendant ever speaking to me during the entire trip. At one point, the thought occurred to me that I could be bleeding to death while this person just sits there. He never checked the amount of blood loss during the trip. Maybe he was too busy trying to breathe himself.

Upon arrival at the hospital, I was rushed to the OB/GYN unit on the second floor. I remember going into labor and being moved to a labor room. When my doctor arrived on the scene, I asked if he was ordering medicine to stop my labor. To my surprise, he refused to even consider it!

"NO!" he snapped. ***"That medication is far too controversial!"*** In one of the few times that I openly questioned this doctor's judgment, I blurted out, *"You mean having a baby at six months* ***ISN'T CONTROVERSIAL?!"***

He gave no response, and his next instruction was just as shocking as his refusal to provide the requested medication. *"Just turn over on your left side to stop the labor."* I could not believe what I was hearing. This man had the ability to give me medicine that could help stop the premature labor, but instead of using it, he was advising me to turn over onto my left side.

At that moment, a sense of total helplessness overcame me. If I had been able to reach the medicine, I would have tried to administer it myself, controversial or not. After all, this medication was used for other people. Why not me? I was desperate to save this precious life within me, and it seemed like this doctor DID NOT have the same goal.

It became obvious that the choice of treatment I would receive was not up to me. I was not given the medicine to stop my labor, and neither was I given any blood to help replenish the huge amount I had lost. The flow was now diminishing somewhat, but I still continued to lose blood steadily.

The next statement this doctor made hit me like a shotgun blast. He repeated it over and over again during the next several days with no remorse nor compassion whatsoever. Staring me in the face, he declared emphatically,

"If your baby is born now, it CANNOT live!"

What a devastating thing for a woman to hear! If anything could drain all hope from you, a statement like that surely would. Maybe this doctor wasn't aware that each person's words contain life or death. Most of his words were filled with gloom and discouragement. If I was going to draw encouragement from someone, it certainly wasn't coming from him.

Chapter 3

Diagnosis

After being in the labor room a few hours, my labor pains surprisingly subsided, and I was moved to a regular semi-private hospital room. This was in the early morning hours of the day I arrived, Monday. Later that morning, my doctor came to advise me that I was being scheduled for an ultra-sound exam. My first thought was, *"Well, why didn't we do this months ago instead of waiting for a catastrophe?"*

Not long after he left, an attendant came and wheeled my bed to the X-ray department. What an experience! We traveled down a maze of halls until we reached a long corridor lined on both sides with hospital beds, each filled with a person waiting to have a "picture" taken. The sight looked like a scene from a Civil War movie with wounded soldiers lying in every available space. My bed was pushed into the first open spot against a wall and parked there.

When my turn finally came, I was wheeled into an X-ray room where a woman technician generously applied a very cold gel to my stomach and began rolling the tip of a microphone-looking instrument around in the gel. At times, she pressed very firmly into my stomach, which caused a great deal of discomfort. As she moved the instrument around on my stomach, a picture on an overhead monitor screen would change. Sound waves from the instrument were producing a live picture of my tiny baby onto that screen.

At the end of the ultrasound, the technician handed me a

snapshot taken during the exam. It was a picture of my unborn baby. The shot was taken looking down onto the top of my baby's head. This picture gave substance to the tiny infant I was carrying. Now, I could actually see the precious treasure I had grown to love so much and was working so hard to protect. It was as though that woman had handed me the keys to a vault full of gold. What a wonderful gift!

Shortly after the exam was over, I was returned to my room, and the doctor soon came to inform me of the results of the ultrasound. Again, what could he give me but more bad news? The ultrasound had revealed that my baby's placenta was attached in the very bottom portion of my uterus instead of the upper part where it belonged. This condition is called placenta previa, and it is life-threatening.

The placenta is the baby's life source through which blood and nourishment flow from the mother. Since this placenta was attached partially over the opening at the bottom of my uterus, precious life-giving blood was being pumped out of my body instead of recirculating. Up to now, I'd heard a lot of negative things from this doctor, but his next words topped them all. Expressionless, he said, *"With this condition, you could bleed to death in a matter of minutes."*

My face must have shown utter shock, then outrage. I was filled with anger and thoughts that I should have said aloud, but didn't. My mind screamed, ***"WHAT?!! AFTER ALL THESE MONTHS OF ME BLEEDING, YOU NOW TELL ME THAT I COULD HAVE BLED TO DEATH IN MINUTES ANY OF THOSE TIMES!!"*** I was furious that he'd allowed me to continue hemorrhaging month after month without ordering an ultrasound to find the cause.

In his familiar monotone voice, he further explained that I would be staying in the hospital totally bedfast until the birth of this child. Not only would I be bedfast, he declared, but the head of my bed could not be raised above the slightest incline. Placenta previa is a very, VERY dangerous condition, and every precaution should be taken to prevent the placenta from dislodging. Why in the world had he waited so long to diagnose this critical problem?! My symptoms had existed for months.

As a side note here, remember the car wreck and heat therapy treatments that I was receiving during the same time frame that I first became pregnant? It is very possible and highly likely that the heat treatments on my lower back may have caused the placenta to dislodge from the upper portion of my uterus. Then, just prior to leaving my body, the placenta could have reattached.

Another possible explanation is that the placenta wasn't ever able to attach in the upper portion of my uterus at all because of the heat therapy treatments. Instead, it may have barely attached at the lowest point just before being completely flushed from my body. Either way, the fact that I had carried this baby for almost six months in such a dangerous condition without miscarrying or bleeding to death was nothing short of a miracle.

The news that I was now being totally confined to bed for the duration of my pregnancy was devastating. But, the next revelation I received brought me a nice bit of comfort in the midst of this storm. A kind-hearted nurse informed me that I could have visits from my young son, Jeremy, since I would be bedfast in the hospital for such a long time. Normally, visitors had to be 12 years of age or older, but an exception was being made, because my hospital stay could potentially be three months long.

The mere thought of now seeing my little boy brought a welcome glimmer of hope into my world. Sadly, someone was standing ready to extinguish the light of that hope during my son's very first visit.

When he walked into my room on the day of his visit, I was elated! I needed a hug from my baby boy, and he needed one from me. This whole ordeal had been very frightening for him, and it was now so reassuring for him to see that I was okay.

But, something had happened since that day the "caring" nurse had given me permission for Jeremy to visit. In fact, she had been replaced by "Hitler's sister" who walked into my room shortly after Jeremy arrived. When she saw a little boy next to my bed, her eyes got as big as saucers.

She gasped for breath and ranted at the top of her lungs, ***"WHAT'S THIS CHILD DOING IN HERE?!! HE'S NOT SUPPOSED TO BE ON THIS FLOOR!!"*** Everyone in the room froze in terror. Instantly, the dam that had been holding back my emotions collapsed. A river of tears began. This woman's calloused, hysterical reaction to seeing my son in my room was the straw that broke the camel's back.

Her dogmatic outburst meant that I would not be able to see Jeremy for the entire duration of my hospital stay, possibly three whole months! That thought was unbearable to me, and nothing could hold back the flood of tears. I cried so hard that my entire body shook. It was obvious that this was traumatizing my already-weakened, hemorrhaging body. The huge strain I was under had finally taken its toll, and this explosion of emotions was the result.

My husband immediately stormed from the room to find my doctor. That was probably not a very good idea. After all, this doctor didn't have a very satisfactory track record of dispensing helpful remedies in tough circumstances. Sure enough, instead of diffusing the tense situation, he fanned the flames when he got there. Upon entering my room and seeing me crying, he glared and said in a disgusted tone, ***"You just need to get ahold of yourself!!"***

Really?!! Let's stand back and do an evaluation of this whole ordeal. Here is a woman who has just recently been told that she has a condition in which she could bleed to death in three minutes. Due to this condition, she has now been restricted to a hospital bed for up to three months. She's lost massive amounts of blood in this pregnancy, and she's repeatedly been bombarded with the news that she will probably lose the unborn child she is carrying.

She has now been informed by a ranting nurse that her four-year-old son is not welcome to visit, even though a previous nurse said he could. Would any sane person think it was strange that this woman was upset and crying?

At that moment, I felt completely helpless and thoroughly assaulted by this doctor's rebuke. I knew that I MUST have some immediate relief from this weight of stress I was under, so I glared back and told him that I wanted to be moved to a private room... RIGHT AWAY!

I felt so sorry that my roommate, Vicki, who was being subjected to this ordeal. She shouldn't have been forced to deal with this stress on top of her own. After all, she was in a very serious condition, as well.

Vicki had previously lost several babies by not being able to carry any of them to full term. Her former doctor had done nothing heroic to help her during the previous pregnancies. Her current doctor, however, was doing everything in his power to help her deliver a miracle this time. He was one of the most caring, concerned physicians I had ever seen, and I was amazed at the excellent care Vicki was receiving. In a way, I hated to leave her company, but I was desperate for the solace that a private room could offer.

My move took place within a few hours. Once I was situated in the new room, a surprising reversal of the "rule" took place. It seems that someone who was higher in authority than "Hitler's sister" had now decided that Jeremy COULD come to visit me after all! My doctor even decided to write an order for my move to the private room, so that my insurance company would cover the entire cost. I was stunned.

During my time in the private room, several things took place. Some are just foggy memories, since I slept much of the time due to blood loss and weakness. One incident, though, stands out vividly. It was the day that a nurse came through the door of my room with a newborn infant in her arms. She walked to the side of my bed and extended the sweetly-wrapped newborn toward me as she proudly said, *"Here's your baby, honey."*

I could hardly believe what I was seeing and hearing. Can you imagine how disheartening this was for me? I was lying flat in bed, having been told repeatedly that my baby probably WOULD NOT live. Now, a nurse is handing me someone else's newborn, thinking it's mine. Bewilderment and sadness both hit me at the same time. I wondered how in the world such a heartbreaking mistake could have ever been made.

When I informed the nurse that I was totally bedfast and had not even HAD my baby yet, all the color drained from her face. She froze when she realized she was handing someone else's baby to a total stranger, a high-risk patient who might never leave the hospital with a living baby. She apologized profusely and backed out the door, protectively clutching her bundle tightly. I will NEVER forget that day!

The one event, though, that totally eclipsed all other memories made in that room was the day my mother came. It was the third or fourth day of my hospitalization. Mom could not visit often, because she was taking care of Jeremy during my hospital stay. As a matter of fact, she only made it there this one time. The powerful impact of this one visit, though, carried me through the remainder of the traumatic ordeal I would have to endure.

Mom was aware that I had continued to bleed and pass clots on a regular basis while hospitalized. She also knew that I had never been given any blood transfusions. When she arrived in my room, she pulled up a chair, sat down by my bed, and opened the book she had brought with her. It was her closest friend. It was her Bible.

She opened its pages, turned to Ezekiel 16:6, and began to read aloud from that precious book:

"And when I passed by thee and saw thee polluted in thine own blood, I said unto thee when thou was in thy blood, 'Live,' yea, I said unto thee when thou was in thy blood, 'Live.' "

When my mom read that powerful verse from the Word of God that day, something unseen but very real happened in my room. A mighty presence filled the place, and I knew without a doubt that I was going to live and that everything was going to be alright!

Chapter 4

Labor & Birth

From the time I arrived at the hospital in the early hours of Monday, May 25, I had consistently gone into labor every other night like clockwork, usually after midnight. Each time this happened, I was moved to a labor room, and the nurses called my doctor. When he showed up, his prescription for me was always the same. *"Turn over on your left side."* My labor usually lasted a few hours before it subsided. I would be returned to my room after the contractions had stopped entirely. Due to the frequency of my labor, I was kept on a liquid diet to prevent complications should a delivery be imminent. Well, imminent it would prove to be.

A little less than five full days after my admittance there, my doctor appeared at the door of my room Friday evening to inform me that he was taking off for the weekend. I could see in his eyes that he was totally exhausted, and I knew my situation was partly to blame, although not through my choice. What I didn't know at the time was that my doctor's decision to leave for the weekend may have been the very thing that saved my baby's life.

My doctor explained that another physician (who I'll call Dr. Williams) would be taking care of me over the weekend. The thought went through my head, *"But I've never even MET this Dr. Williams! I'm in a life-threatening condition, and you're leaving me in the hands of a total stranger?!"* It felt like I was being abandoned mid-stream, but in actuality, God was working things for my good! Poof! Bad doc gone.

As surely as the sun comes up in the East and sets in the

West, I went into labor again. This time, it was around 1 AM on Saturday morning, and it meant another trip to the labor room down the hall. However, this trip was going to be completely different from all the others.

The nurses called Dr. Williams who showed up immediately. From the first moment I laid eyes on this man in the wee hours of that morning, I knew that he had been sent by God. He was an older, white-haired gentleman with the kindest eyes and smile you could ever imagine. I remember how he introduced himself to me and shook my hand. He then turned to a nurse and proceeded to pour out directions for my care. I could hardly believe my ears. He was actually ordering medical treatment for my labor!

Dr. Williams obviously had two priorities. The first was to stop my labor, and the second was to replenish my blood. He quickly ordered an intravenous solution of the controversial medication that my regular doctor had refused to give me. Imagine my surprise and relief upon hearing that.

Next, he ordered a blood transfusion for me. I was so overwhelmed by this man's concern for me that tears came into my eyes. Finally, someone was in charge who seemed to actually care about helping my baby and me. When Dr. Williams saw my tears, he walked to the side of my bed and gently patted my hand. He told me that he intended to do everything in his power to help me. At that moment, I felt like I was looking at an angel in doctors' clothing.

A nurse hurried into the room to start an IV of the labor-stopping medication, ritodrine. From the moment this drug hit my bloodstream, everything in my body instantly went into high speed. Within just a few minutes of receiving the med, I quickly understood why controversy surrounded it. My heart rate skyrocketed unbelievably, and I could feel my heart pounding like a jackhammer in my head and ears. It was similar to a small airplane trying to take off inside me. I remember thinking at one point that I could possibly have a stroke or might even die.

One important point to remember: this medication not only caused MY heart rate to soar, but it also affected my unborn baby's heart in the very same way. I would later learn that my baby benefitted from the stress that this med put on her heart and metabolism. Both were strengthened and exercised by the stress.

The impact of ritodrine on my body was so dramatic that I needed round-the-clock monitoring while I was on this IV. A nurse was posted beside my bed to constantly watch my heart rate and blood pressure. She didn't leave my side all day unless another nurse came to relieve her. Most of the time, she didn't even need to touch my wrist or neck to take my pulse. She simply counted the beats she saw as the arteries in my neck pulsated intensely.

The exhausting stress continued until early afternoon. By that time, I was totally drained physically and was extremely thirsty. I begged for something to drink, but the only thing I could have in my mouth was one of those nasty spearmint-flavored swabs. I fully understood that it was very important to keep my stomach empty in case I should need an anesthetic, but that knowledge did nothing to ease my thirst.

Other monitoring of my condition was also taking place. Whenever a woman is in labor in this hospital, two narrow belts are placed around her stomach area. Each one contains a sensitive device that sends data to a machine beside the bed. One belt measures the severity of labor contractions, while the other belt measures the baby's heartbeat. This crucial data gives the medical team vital information about the advancement of labor and the baby's well being.

One unique problem that presented itself in my case was my baby's small size at this stage of development. If the baby moved into a different section of my stomach away from the belt, the monitor couldn't pick up the heart rate. When that happened, the machine registered no heartbeat at all. This was cause for major panic among the medical personnel in the room, since it could be an indicator that the infant was in distress. Each time they finally relocated my baby, the heart belt had to be readjusted on my stomach. This happened over and over again through the day. After a bit, the nurses decided that my baby must have created its own version of the game Hide and Seek, and the baby was definitely winning.

During those times when the belt was properly picking up the heartbeat, the nurses tried to guess whether the baby was a boy or a girl based on the heart rate. A boy's rate is normally faster than a girl's, so they leaned toward the opinion that it was probably a boy. But, they also knew that the medication was dramatically spiking the heart rate, so they didn't put a lot of confidence in their decision.

Throughout the entire day, I was constantly trying to find a comfortable position in which to lie. It was impossible. There just wasn't one. I had used up all my options very early in the morning. It was extremely painful for my knees to touch each other when I turned onto my side. So, a kind nurse brought me a pillow to put between my knees. That might seem like such an insignificant thing to some people, but I still remember that kindness to this day.

By mid-afternoon, my labor totally stopped. That was a real cause for rejoicing, but I didn't have much strength to do any celebrating. I was finally disconnected from the IV containing the ritodrine, but the other IV was left intact in case I needed more blood to replenish what I continued to lose. It was decided that I should remain in the labor room a little longer, just as a precaution.

There was such compassion in Dr. William's face as he gently patted my hand and said, *"My Dear, if you make it to 7 o'clock tonight without any more labor pains, you can go back to your room and have a cold soft drink!"* He might just as well have said that I could have a million dollars, because an ice cold soft drink was exactly what I wanted at that time. Unfortunately, I would not be getting the desired soft drink anytime soon. Matter of fact, it would be quite some time before I could even return to my own room at all.

Shortly before the deadline of 7 PM, my labor pains started again. The doctor decided that I should not be put back on ritodrine, because of the toll it had taken on my body already. He felt it would be unwise to restart it. So, we were now back in the labor stage again.

As I've said, my baby had repeatedly dodged the heart monitor strapped to my stomach. This kept everyone so busy trying to locate the baby that no one noticed the serious problem that had developed with the OTHER belt.

Unknown to anyone in the room, the monitor on the second belt was not accurately picking up the intensity of my labor contractions. This belt had been placed on the upper part of my stomach in the normal position for someone with a full-term pregnancy. However, my tiny baby was not positioned in the upper half of my abdomen where that belt was placed. My baby was in the lowest part of my abdomen, and my uterus was much smaller due to this pregnancy's short term. Therefore, the belt was sitting much too high to accurately record the true intensity of the contractions that were taking place in the lower quadrant of my stomach. No one really knew just how far I was into labor because of the weak signals they were reading.

But, I was becoming more and more aware that my pains had intensified dramatically and were getting much closer together. So, I shared this information with the next nurse who came into my room. She took a look at the reading on the bedside machine, then assured me there was nothing to be concerned about and left the room, not knowing that the belt wasn't in a proper position to accurately gauge my labor.

Not long after that, I buzzed the desk and asked to have a nurse come to my room. When one arrived, I tried to explain exactly what I was feeling. The monitor was consulted by this nurse, and I was again assured that everything was fine. She also left the room. I am quite sure that my next call moments

later sounded like a frantic 9-1-1 call when I shouted,
"I FEEL LIKE I'M HAVING THIS BABY RIGHT NOW!!"

Immediately, two nurses came running into my room. One of them moved the contraction belt to a new position on my stomach. When it settled on the lower portion of my abdomen, the reading on the machine pegged to the top of the scale! This nurse's face went ashen as she gasped,
"OH MY GOSH! WE'D BETTER CALL DR. WILLIAMS!!"

He must have already been in the hospital when he got the emergency call, because he was in my room within minutes examining me. He quickly turned to a nurse and stressed an order, ***"Get her to the delivery room NOW!!"***

When I heard those words, I had a sudden flashback to something my regular doctor had told me multiple times here in the hospital. He had repeatedly said, *"With placenta previa, you MUST have a cesarean delivery, or your baby will be born dead. With a natural birth, the placenta would be delivered first, cutting off your baby's lifeline."* But, it didn't sound like Dr. Williams was planning to do a cesarean!!?

With alarm in my voice, I said, *"Dr. Williams, my other doctor said I have to have a cesarean delivery or the placenta will come first, and my baby will be born dead!"* Again, this precious man who was sent by God patted my hand and reassured me. He calmly said, *"Honey it's going to be alright. Your baby has somehow gone around the placenta. When I examined you just now, I saw your baby's head."*

With those words, an amazing peace invaded the room. You could literally feel it. A calm that words cannot describe descended on all of us there, and a hush fell over the room. We were witnessing the grace, protection, and provision of God in the middle of a storm.

Suddenly, my bed and I were both being rushed from the labor room, down the hall, and into the delivery room. Since my son had been born in this hospital four years earlier,

I was somewhat familiar with the delivery procedure. However, some things had changed in those four years. For one thing, the father could now be present during the delivery. At Jeremy's birth, even the labor room had been off limits to everyone except me.

Now, a nurse was hurrying my husband into a side room to quickly scrub his hands and don a hospital gown over his clothes. It was at this point that I found myself alone in the delivery room with that one solitary nurse.

Just then, I felt an uncontrollable urge to push with all my might. Through clinched teeth, I relayed that serious bit of information to my single sentry nurse. Panic filled her eyes as she gasped and pleaded, *"Please, DON'T push! Whatever you do, just DON'T push!"* It was at this point she leaned as close to the open door as possible, without leaving my side, and pressed the panic button with her voice.

> ***"HELP! ... SOMEONE HELP!!***
> ***SOMEONE, PLEASE HELP!!"***

Suddenly, the room was filled with those eight or nine doctors and nurses that I mentioned at the beginning of this book. They arrived not a minute too soon. There was no time for delay. They barely got into place, and within mere seconds, the baby was here!

As soon as my baby was born, Dr. Williams made the most precious announcement I could have hoped to hear. With my tiny baby in his cradled hands, he exhaled gently and said in his wonderful, loving tone, *"Ohhhhhhh look! It's a little baby girl!"* My heart leaped. A baby girl! Exactly what I'd wanted. Instantly, I was overwhelmed with gratitude for God and for Dr. Williams.

Only the briefest glance of my newborn daughter was possible as she was whisked into the waiting arms of the perinatal center crew. There was no time for me to bond with my precious child. Her life was hanging in the balance.

Just before Dr. Williams handed her to the specialists, though, a most amazing thing happened. My tiny baby girl opened her little mouth and started to cry! It was both beautiful and astonishing. Here was a baby whose lungs could not possibly be fully developed at a gestation of 26 weeks, and yet, she was crying out with her own little tiny voice, and I heard it!

I cannot adequately describe for you what that one simple sound did for me. At the exact moment that my baby cried, something remarkable happened. A special gift directly from God was suddenly imparted to me to help carry me through the difficult days that were ahead.

I was receiving the gift of "unmovable faith" talked about in First Corinthians 12: 4-11. I literally felt it settle down inside me, and I boldly said within myself,

"If this baby is strong enough to cry,
she's strong enough to make it!"

From that moment on, NO ONE would be able to convince me that my baby would not survive and be perfectly fine. So, on May 30, 1981, a miracle was born at 9:33 PM!

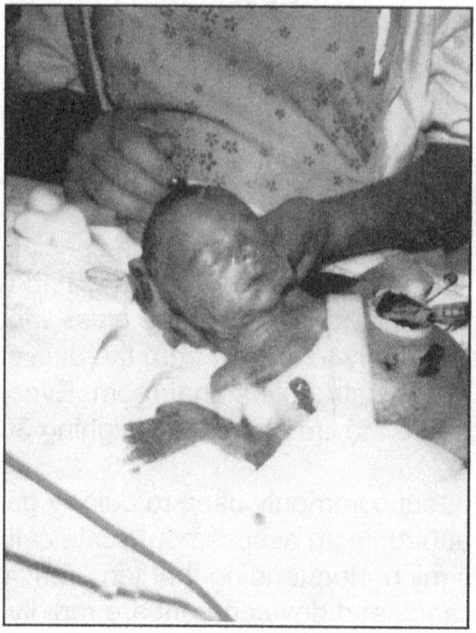

- Seven days old -

To accurately gauge her size, note the cotton ball on her right arm and the safety pin near her left one.

Chapter 5

Critical

Within moments of my baby's birth, the specialists were working feverishly to help her survive. They had whisked her into a small adjoining room with a large glass window. If I turned my head sharply to the left from the delivery table, I could see the intense struggle in that room. Every effort was being made to save the life of a baby weighing 30 ounces.

One valuable tool commonly used to quickly gauge a baby's health at birth is an assessment scale called the Apgar test. It is my understanding that ten areas of the infant's appearance and development are rapidly analyzed and scored. Each of these ten areas are assigned one point. So, if a baby is born normal and healthy, it should easily attain a score of ten using the Apgar method.

I'd never heard of the Apgar test at that time, and it's probably a good thing that no one mentioned it to me. If they had, it might have brought a great deal of fear my way, since my baby's score immediately following her birth was extremely low. I would later discover that she only scored a THREE!

While all of this analyzing and activity was taking place in my delivery room, something equally as dramatic was happening just a few doors away. Unknown to me, only moments after the crucial phone call had reached the perinatal center requesting an emergency team of medical specialists for my baby's birth, a second call came there urgently requesting ANOTHER team of perinatal center specialists ASAP!

A SECOND premature delivery was taking place only a few paces down the hall from me!

Believe it or not, this second team was needed at the same time for the birth of my former roommate's baby. Shockingly, Vicki was delivering her baby three months prematurely just like me! Only nine minutes after my baby was born, Vicki's daughter made her grand entrance into the world weighing even less. These two back-to-back dramatic births practically emptied the perinatal center of specialists and technicians for a good while.

(The memory of this night still lives vividly in the minds of some doctors and nurses who were working that shift in 1981. I was privileged to speak with a few of them years later when Vicki and I returned with our daughters to the perinatal center on the day the girls turned ten years old.)

Not long after my baby's birth, I was moved from the delivery room back to the very same labor room where I had just spent the most eventful day of my entire life. It was at this time that I learned Dr. Williams had earlier taken my husband into the hall to ask him a very serious question. *"If worse comes to worse, and we are faced with a decision, should we try to save your wife's life or your unborn baby's life?"*

When I found out that a life-or-death decision about MY life was laid in my husband's lap instead of mine, I was shocked! After all, I wasn't unconscious or delirious when the question was posed to my husband, so why wasn't I asked? This was a decision about MY LIFE, not my husband's. Upon hearing about the discussion, I was stunned and disturbed that I had never been consulted, when I was the one who had the most to gain or lose from the decision.

As I lay there in that familiar labor room once again, the harsh reality of what had just taken place began to pressure my mind. I had just given birth to a baby who had the odds tremendously stacked against her. She was born three full months earlier than she should have been, and things did not look good for her. From somewhere outside of me, negative thoughts began to rapidly hit my mind like machine gun bullets. *"What if she doesn't make it? She's so tiny! How can she possibly live? What if she dies? What are you going to do?* ***What in the world are you going to do?!"***

Right in the middle of the onslaught of oppressive thoughts, a nurse hurriedly rushed into my room as though she was looking for the answer to the 64-million-dollar question. *"Honey,"* she quickly asked, *"Are you going to breast feed?"*

"Huh??" I wondered to myself. *"Doesn't she know they aren't even sure if my baby will survive?"* But, another thought then came. *"Wait a minute! Maybe something has changed. She wants to know if I'm going to breast feed, so maybe they now think my baby IS going to make it!"* My face brightened, and hope suddenly began to rise.

"Well, uh ... Yes! ... ***YES!"*** was my response. At the time, I had no idea they were simply asking that question in order to determine if I needed an injection of medicine to prevent lactation, since the shot has to be given shortly after birth. I thought they were asking because they believed my baby was going to pull through now. Regardless of their reason for asking that question, it came at exactly the right time to help bolster my faith, and that's exactly what it did.

By this time, not far from me on the same hospital floor, a whole new ball game had begun for my baby. She'd been thrust from a warm, safe, protected environment that should have been her home for another three months. From there, she'd landed in a cold, harsh battle for her life. She was now in a setting that required her to be kept fairly isolated, even from those who loved her the most. But, survival was the name of the game that this baby was now struggling to win.

A few hours after giving birth, I was taken back to my room. Even though I was totally exhausted and needed rest, I was anxious to see my new baby girl, since I'd never even gotten to take a close look at her yet. Shortly after arriving at my room, I asked to be allowed to go to the intensive care nursery to see my baby. It did not matter to me that it was still in the wee hours of the morning.

The nurse I asked was so compassionate that she gladly helped me don my robe and slippers for this trip of a lifetime. A wheelchair was my limousine, since I was much too weak to walk the long distance to the perinatal center on my own. We traveled down a maze of hallways and turns before my chauffeur-driven vehicle pulled up to a big glass window, then stopped. I slowly stood to my feet and was absolutely shocked at what I saw. It looked like a miniature city behind that huge pane of glass.

Even at this late hour of the night, the place was lit up like an underground parking garage. Everywhere you looked were rows and rows of tiny beds side-by-side. These beds were unlike any baby bed I had ever seen before. They looked more like some kind of space-age beds. My former perception of an incubator disintegrated as I viewed these modern marvels.

Each bed was narrow and consisted of a flat, elevated platform about 3 - 4 feet from the floor. That rectangular section created the mattress portion and wasn't more than two feet wide and maybe 3 feet long. The side railings were six-inch-tall glass panels to prevent the babies from rolling out. Most of the babies I saw, however, looked like they could barely move, much less roll out of the bed. Truth is, many of them looked like they were barely alive.

Approximately two feet above the platform mattress on each bed was a metal cover containing lights and a heating element that served to help warm the baby. On many of the beds, these lights were rarely ever turned off, unless the infant occupying that bed passed away.

There in the midst of that sterile city of modern incubators lay the tiniest baby I'd ever seen. I was shocked to find out it was MY baby! She seemed to be the smallest baby there.

Her bed was at the end of a row, and she was far enough away from the window that I couldn't get a really good look at her. I wanted to be closer to her, but the nurse who had wheeled me there was already gone now, and I'd not been informed of the proper procedure to be admitted into the perinatal center. So, I had to be content with just standing there on the outside looking into my baby's new world.

After several minutes, my limited strength ran out, and I needed to return to my room. Even though I was excited to finally see my tiny baby girl, my body was too drained to handle more.

My husband wheeled my "limousine" back to the room. When it pulled up beside my bed, I gladly crawled under the covers knowing that I would NOT be going to a labor room again. That part of this journey was over. Sleep settled in for the first time in more than 24 hours.

Chapter 6

Preemie

Around 8 AM, I was awakened by a middle-aged woman with a clipboard in her hands. She smiled pleasantly as she entered my room, and I wondered why she was there. *"Have you decided on a name for your baby?"* she cheerfully asked. Apparently, she was in charge of collecting name data on newborns.

As I opened my mouth to tell her the name I'd chosen, a horrible thought suddenly shot into my mind. It was almost as though an audible voice whispered ominously, *"Don't waste your favorite name. Your baby is going to die."* The voice seemed so real that I almost looked around to see who had spoken.

But, as quickly as that horrible thought had come, something bigger rose up on the inside of me to drive it out. It was FAITH! I heard faith coming from my mouth boldly telling this census-taking lady, *"Yes, I DO have a name picked out. It's my favorite name. My baby's name is Janessa Lynn."*

When I spoke those words, it was like fire fell from Heaven and totally consumed the fear that had previously delivered doubt to my mind. The data lady proudly documented my choice on her clipboard, smiled, and thanked me. She then moved to another room. I was quickly learning that faith had something to say, and I needed to be saying it.

Not long after that incident, my first set of visitors arrived. I really was not feeling much like having company yet, but an aunt and uncle by marriage had just learned about the premature birth and obviously hurried down to see what a baby who weighs only 30 ounces looks like.

Slowly, I led the way to the intensive care nursery. It was a slower trip this time, because I was walking instead of using a wheelchair. We made our way down the long hallways to the very same glass window I had visited during the night. Not a thing had changed on the other side of the glass. It was still as bright as ever. Even though there were no exterior windows that I could see in the unit, it stayed intensely bright around the clock.

Research now shows that it's better to lessen the harshness of lights for premature babies in a critical-care facility. This information was obviously not available at the time my baby was there, however, because every light in the place was brightly lit continuously.

These visiting relatives behaved like people at a circus sideshow. They didn't even try to hide their shock and disbelief when they saw Janessa lying in that incubator. If she had been a typical full-term baby, the sounds coming from their mouths would have been soft forms of *"oooooooo" or "ooohhhhhh."* But instead, these two people loudly blurted, ***"OOOOOOHHHHHHH MYYYYYYY GOSH!!"*** *and* ***"OOOOOOOHHHHHHH HOW SAD!!"***

I don't mind telling you that a little of that went a long way with me, and I was ready very quickly to return to my room and bid these two goodbye. Thoughts were racing in and out of my head. *"If they can't say anything positive, why don't they just keep their mouths shut?!"* It was at this point I acknowledged to myself that they obviously didn't come to encourage and support me. They had only come to see something they had never seen before. It truly WAS a sideshow to them, just like a circus, except they didn't have to pay to see this one. I did.

We came back to my room, and they finally left. Their presence had been very draining to me emotionally, so I really wasn't sorry to see them go. Right after they left, in their place came a nice person selling newspapers door-to-door. I've always liked to read, so I bought one with some change from the top drawer of my nightstand. Even though I knew it was much too soon for my baby's birth announcement to be listed in the vital statistics section, I still turned to that page. I scanned the names. Nope, not there yet.

I was starting a daily routine of looking. Unfortunately, my routine would turn up nothing day after day. Several days passed with no results, so I called the newspaper office to ask when my baby's birth would be announced. The answer I got was a full-blown "slap in the face" to my faith.

The newspaper lady on the other end of the line told me their paper never prints the birth of a baby who goes straight into an intensive care nursery, because so many of those babies do not survive. Unbelievable! When I got that answer, red hot anger flared up in me. What a negative approach for a newspaper to take.

Righteous indignation rose up in me due to the "inside information" that I had in my spirit. I boldly informed the lady on the phone that she needed to get a pen and paper to take down my baby's information, because it DEFINITELY was going to be printed in their newspaper.

I was beginning to better understand that it would require serious determination on my part to maintain the faith that had been delivered to me. Around every corner lurked some-one with a negative comment or some bad news. But, the ball was in MY court. The final decision was mine. Whose report would I choose to believe?

When a nurse stepped into my room to check on me, I asked when I would be allowed to touch my new baby. Com-passion came bubbling up from this sweet lady who knew my baby had likely been whisked from my sight at birth. She graciously gave me clear instructions on where and how to enter the sterile perinatal center and told me that someone there would direct me further. Finally! I was actually going to be able to touch my baby girl.

Carefully following the nurse's directions, I hurried down the maze of hallways to the perinatal center and waited at the open doorway. No one came right away, and it was several minutes before anyone in the unit noticed me. Since there were probably 40 critical-care infants there at the time, it was completely understandable that the nurses were all extremely busy. When I was finally spotted, a kindhearted nurse came to show me the proper procedure for entering the "world of the sterile" where Janessa now lived.

The nurse pointed to my right, just inside the doorway. There was a fairly small, closet-like space with two very deep metal sinks. Adjacent to the sinks was a large metal rack with shelves that reached to the ceiling. Each shelf contained stacks of neatly folded, freshly laundered hospital gowns. My new instructions were to first put a hospital gown over my clothing and then step to the sinks, which I did.

To the left of the sinks was a huge cardboard box holding hundreds of individually wrapped plastic packages that each contained a small scrub brush. On the back ledge of each sink was a large bottle of brownish-colored disinfectant soap. I was now supposed to scrub my hands and fingernails with the brush and soap for three full minutes.

Three minutes of hand washing seemed like an eternity. A line of people formed behind me and also beside me at the next sink. All of them were parents anxious to rid themselves of their germs in order to gain entrance into the sterile environment that was home to their babies.

When I had scrubbed until my hands resembled prunes, I stepped for the first time into the massive room that I'd previously only viewed through that large pane of glass. A wonderful nurse led the way to Janessa's area. As I approached her bed and saw her up close for the very first time, I was overwhelmed and ached to do something to help my baby.

As I looked at her tiny, yellow, wrinkled body, I thought to myself, *"Oh my gosh! She looks dead!"*

A machine was providing oxygen and was mechanically breathing for her through a tube inserted in her mouth. One of her tiny arms was taped tightly to a tongue depressor to keep that arm immobile so an IV needle would not dislodge. The tape was pulled so tightly that it dented into her arm. It looked to me like it would surely cut off her circulation. My first instinct as a mother was to loosen the tape immediately, but I knew better. Little did I know that this troubling sight was only the first of many painful things I would observe.

On her chest was a silver-colored electrode approximately the size of a half-dollar coin. It was attached to her body with some type of sticky substance. This electrode measured the level of oxygen in her skin. That figure was then used to tell the breathing machine how much oxygen to supply. If her skin wasn't receiving enough oxygen, that meant her vital organs weren't either. If the reading was too low, the percentage of oxygen supplied would be increased.

Here lay this tiny, naked, wrinkled, yellowish-colored baby on a newborn disposable diaper that was pulled open completely so it would lay flat. It absolutely swallowed her tiny body. In comparison, looking at her on this small newborn diaper was like looking at a full-term baby on a receiving blanket.

While standing beside her bed, I turned to glance around the room. Imagine my shock when I saw a familiar face on the next row just across the aisle! It was Dwight, a man who lived next door to my aunt and uncle in the town from which I'd just moved. He was standing by the bed of his new baby, Michelle, who had been born only a few days earlier in the town where I now lived. Since I rarely ever saw him and his wife, I had no idea they were even expecting a baby.

Their baby had been transferred to this hospital's perinatal center in a specially equipped vehicle that was specifically designed for transporting critical infants. Michelle was a full-term, full-sized newborn, but she had some major issues.

Doctors were unsure exactly what was wrong with Michelle, but they strongly suspected that her heart was somehow hooked up backwards. They had no idea how she had lived these few days since her birth. Emergency plans were being made to airlift her to a special children's hospital in our state, if time did not run out for her first. I spoke with Dwight and found out that his wife was still hospitalized in my new home-town. All of this was very hard for them, especially his wife, since she was not even in the same hospital as Michelle and could not see nor touch her baby.

As I walked back to my own baby's bed, a horrible thought crept into my mind. *"Their baby is much bigger and healthier-looking than Janessa, but the doctors don't give them much hope at all. What makes you think Janessa will make it, since she already looks dead?!"*

The stark reality of that statement was staring me in the face as I looked down at the pitiful condition of Janessa's tiny body. But, instead of meditating on that awful possibility, I quickly went back in my memory to the moment when she was born.

I remembered the rock-solid peace that had settled into my spirit when I first heard her cry. I remembered the confidence that had anchored inside me at that moment. I remembered about FAITH!

So, instead of bowing to the present assault on my faith, I said, *"No, Mr. Devil. I'm not buying the lie you just sent me. My baby IS going to make it? She IS going to live!"* Instantly, that oppression left me. It was like I had stomped my foot and shouted, *"SCAT!"* That negative thought was gone as quickly as it had come.

When the nurse returned, I began asking some questions about Janessa's condition and prognosis. Since this woman had worked with these situations, I wanted her thoughts and perspective. Her guarded responses, however, told me that she was extremely reluctant to discuss anything about Janessa's case with me.

As time went on, I would discover that most medical professionals are hesitant to tell you anything that might "get your hopes up" or "give you false hope" in this type of situation. As a matter of fact, it often seems like they feel it necessary to give you only the "down side" of what to expect.

Throughout this lengthy ordeal, I would learn by experience that I was basically on my own with my "expect-and-believe-the-best" attitude. There would be very few people willing to join me over on the FAITH SIDE.

Chapter 7

Negative Reports

During the time I was in the hospital recuperating, it was comforting to be able to visit Janessa often. The day quickly came, however, for me to be dismissed. That meant I had to leave my precious baby behind. Even though I had carried her in, I would not be carrying her out ... at least not yet.

So, on the bittersweet morning that I was released from the hospital, I cried as I bent down to kiss Janessa goodbye. A very familiar feeling rushed over me at that moment. This was my second child born alive, and it was now the second time I would be leaving the hospital without my newborn baby.

Four years earlier, Jeremy's severe case of jaundice at birth kept him hospitalized for five days, while I was forced to leave on the third day. But, those few days of separation from him would pale in comparison to what lay ahead now. I had no idea exactly how long this journey would be, but I did know that I would be returning to the hospital again and again until the day I could finally bring my baby girl home with me. After carefully kissing her tiny face, I slowly turned from her bed and left the hospital with tears in my eyes, having never even gotten to hold her in my arms yet.

I went home, but my absence from the hospital did not last long. Less than 24 hours later, I was back there standing beside Janessa's bed again. To be able to return to the hospital, it had been necessary for me to drive my husband 17 miles to work early in the morning so that I could use our only car. The hospital was about seven miles from his job. It was around 8 AM when I pulled into the parking lot. This was starting a routine that I would follow day after day for a very long time.

On one particular day, a real shock awaited me when I arrived upstairs. I parked the car, proceeded to the peri-natal center, sterilized my hands, and then headed in Janessa's direction. Just as I reached her bed, a horrendous noise started blaring from the panel above her. It resembled a freightliner's horn blowing.

Immediately, a nurse rushed to the bedside, scanned the monitor mounted at the head of the bed, pushed a button to silence the alarm, then quickly picked up one of Janessa's little feet. With the thumb and first finger of her right hand, this nurse began forcefully thumping the bottom of that tiny foot that measured barely over an inch long.

I had no idea what was happening. I did not know that Janessa had completely stopped breathing. The alarm had signaled it, and this nurse was now attempting to shock Janessa into breathing again. With her finger, she flipped the bottom of that little foot relatively hard again and again while I stood watching in stunned disbelief.

About 30 seconds later, Janessa was roused into breathing again. But, it certainly took more than 30 seconds for my heart to settle down. This would prove to be my crash course in heroic life-saving techniques for premature babies. Sure wish I would have been given advance warning!

After spending a few hours at the hospital, I needed to head for home. I wanted to be with Jeremy and also get some things done around the house before going to pick up my husband from work. I'd missed Jeremy so much, and he needed my attention. After all, I'd been gone over a week. So, I drove home, and he and I got to have a good time together before I dropped him off at my mom's house again. Next stop was to pick up my husband and go back to the hospital for the evening. This would become part of my regular routine for the next three months.

When I'd made a number of these trips back and forth to the hospital, I started getting concerned that no doctor had spoken with me about Janessa's condition. My only contact with medical personnel had been with the various nurses who were attending Janessa. They all seemed to be seriously limited in what information they could give me. This was very frustrating, so I began asking to speak to a doctor.

It seemed odd to me that I was forced to request a meeting with a doctor, given the graveness of the situation. I thought a doctor should have been asking to meet with me. After I made my request, it took a few days for the meeting to be arranged, but appointment time finally came.

My husband and I were shuffled into a small, closet-like room just outside the perinatal center. The tiny space contained very little in the way of furnishings. It only had a desk and chair for the doctor, plus two small chairs for my husband and I. Due to the tiny space, the other medical person present was forced to squeeze beside the doctor's chair and stand against the wall through the entire meeting.

The doctor (Dr. K) introduced herself in a heavy Greek accent. She had a serious look on her face and a very stern tone in her voice as she began a verbal dissertation of my baby's case. According to her, Janessa had a very, VERY slim chance of survival, probably only ten percent. Additionally, if Janessa DID live, the odds were extremely high that she would have major complications. Some of the words the doctor used were "brain damage, blindness, deafness, intestinal removal, and heart problems," just to name a few.

Dr. K was speaking from years of experience with these types of cases. She was attempting to make it clear to me that there was no hope Janessa could ever be normal. As a matter of fact, Dr. K said she strongly suspected there was blood leakage in Janessa's brain, and Dr. K was ordering a CT scan to confirm that. She further explained that leaking blood in the brain is a strong indicator of brain damage.

Everything Dr. K said in this meeting painted a negative, hopeless picture. She had no way to know that I had inside information coming from a higher source than any that was visible to the natural eye. The calm assurance I had been given at Janessa's birth was carrying me peacefully through this very difficult session.

The whole meeting lasted about 15 minutes, with Dr. K doing all the talking. Near the end, she leaned toward me and glared into my face with a very stern look. It wasn't clear to me what had prompted this behavior in her until she then turned toward my husband and raised her voice in an agitated tone. She firmly said to him, ***"I want you to take your wife home and explain to her everything I've just told you, because she hasn't heard a word I said!"***

Wow! My calm attitude and the peaceful look on my face had apparently angered this doctor and convinced her that I was in total denial and was avoiding the reality of this very serious situation. After she said that to my husband, she immediately stood up in that tiny, crowded space, and the meeting was abruptly over. We all left the room, and she disappeared into her office down the hall.

Words are a mighty powerful force. In the same way that we had followed Dr. K from that closet room, her negative words tried to follow me around the rest of the day. However, the strong faith with which I'd been infused at Janessa's birth rose up to meet the challenge. So, instead of me striking out when the doctor threw that curve ball of negativity at me, the special faith I'd received simply stepped closer to the plate and knocked those words out of the ballpark.

Well, Dr. K obviously took my so-called "denial" very seriously! Upon my arrival at the hospital the next day, I was met by a woman introducing herself as a "caseworker" who had now been assigned to me. This was a total surprise to me. The only caseworkers I'd ever heard of were ones that dealt with people who were "at risk" or on welfare.

This woman talked briefly to me as I stood there. She asked me to submit to a multiple-choice written test that I could take home to complete. I got the strangest feeling that this request was coming as a direct result of the meeting with Dr. K the day before, but I didn't mention that and agreed to take the test.

When looking over the test at home that night, I quickly discovered that it was obviously a psychological evaluation. It contained about 500 questions and was designed in such a way that the same questions were being asked over and over again, with only a slight variation in the wording each time.

I suppose it would be difficult for an unstable or dishonest person to pass the test, since it would be hard to remember exactly how you had answered 500 separate questions. At any rate, I was fairly certain that my calmness and my refusal to respond "appropriately" to Dr. K's bad news had convinced them that I was a person who needed evaluating. I completed the test and turned it in.

Not long after I submitted it, the report from the CT scan of Janessa's brain came back. The report stated there were pools of blood in her brain that indicated a very serious complication. According to Dr. K in our meeting, this was tragically a common problem in premature infants.

At first mention of the alarming CT results, a shock wave rumbled through me. Within minutes, though, that perfect peace I had been experiencing settled over me once again, and a calm returned.

To my surprise, the doctor ordered another CT brain scan not long after this. That seemed unusual to me, and I didn't understand why a repeat scan would be done so soon. When I got the results of the second scan, though, I saw the dramatic effect that faith was having. This next scan found absolutely NO BLOOD pooled in Janessa's brain!

The earlier negative report had completely reversed itself,

and there was no natural explanation as to how that amount of blood had just disappeared and been replaced with brain matter in such a short time. Needless to say, I left the hospital that day on a tremendous high!

A few days later, however, my emotions were assaulted by yet another potentially damaging blow. During my routine visit, I went through the procedure of scrubbing and donning a gown. As usual, I then headed for Janessa's bed. This time, though, as I rounded the corner of her aisle, I noticed several doctors and nurses crowded around the bed next to hers. They were frantically working on the baby who occupied that bed. This infant was much bigger and had seemed so much healthier than Janessa. It was shocking to see this baby now in such distress.

When one of the nurses glanced up and saw me standing at Janessa's bed watching them, she quickly rushed over and asked me to please go downstairs to the coffee shop for a little while. Based on her behavior and the crowd of medical professionals there, I knew this must surely be extremely serious. The urgency in her voice and what I was viewing prompted me to quickly agree, so I left.

I stayed away from the perinatal center about an hour, then returned and went through the sanitizing procedure once again. This time when I rounded Janessa's corner, the sight I saw stopped me in my tracks. The bed next to hers was empty! It was freshly cleaned and dressed with new linens, and the lights on the panel above it were turned off. There was no longer a baby in that bed desperately needing medical intervention from doctors and nurses.

That baby had died while I was downstairs at the coffee shop! I cannot adequately tell you how profoundly I was affected by this devastating loss. I had seen this baby every time I came to visit Janessa. But I would never see it again.

My heart began beating faster and faster, and tears came. A heavy sense of despair almost overwhelmed me. That baby had appeared to be doing so well all along. What could have happened?

Scary thoughts then began to weasel their way into my mind. I looked at Janessa lying there in such a pitiful condition with tubes running into her body and an IV stuck in her head. She had electrodes pasted all over, and she wasn't even half the size of the baby who had just died. What made me think she could possibly survive when other healthier-looking babies were dying? Nausea came creeping in with all those horrible thoughts.

Then, all of a sudden, it felt like somebody bigger than me stood up on the inside. I lifted my head and decided that the other precious baby's tragic death was not going to determine Janessa's outcome. As a matter of fact, I decided to do something substantial just to prove it. Up to this point, I had never been allowed to hold Janessa due to her serious condition. Therefore, I had absolutely no reason to think I would be allowed to do it now. But, I was determined to push back against the fear that was pushing me at present. So, I found a nearby nurse and boldly asked if I could please hold Janessa for the very first time.

To my utter amazement, this precious nurse quickly rushed to accommodate my request by dragging a rocking chair over to the bed. I seated myself while she gathered tubes, lines, and cords into one of her hands. Then, she carefully lifted my tiny 25-ounce baby girl into my waiting arms.

As I held Janessa for the very first time, incredible joy filled my heart. I spoke to her softly and sang to her quietly. She seemed to snuggle down into my arms in precious, peaceful contentment.

The blow I had just experienced through the tragic death of her infant roommate was replaced by the awesome fulfillment that a mother receives when holding her new baby for the very first time. This was a moment of real victory for my faith.

Please excuse the poor quality of these pictures.
They survived a house fire shortly before Janessa's 2nd birthday.
(An undeveloped roll of film was discovered.)

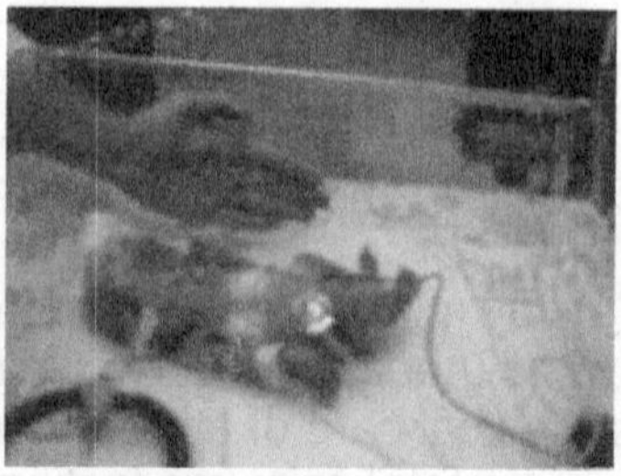

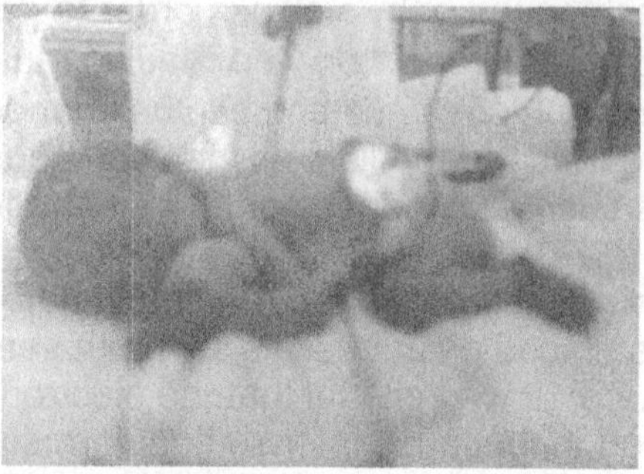

Janessa on an opened-up newborn disposable diaper that looks like a receiving blanket in comparison to her tiny size.

Also note the makeshift pacifier that is actually a cap and nipple from a tiny, preemie-sized baby bottle.

Chapter 8

Circumstances

During Janessa's stay in the perinatal center, I would come to understand firsthand that there's very little room for error when handling the medical care of a premature infant. The slightest mistake can be fatal or cause lasting impairment. Here's an example.

It is extremely important to constantly monitor the amount of oxygen reaching the baby's skin in order to determine the proper setting for the ventilator. The reading must be available every moment, so the setting can be changed quickly if needed. Too much or too little oxygen can cause serious complications such as blindness or brain damage.

To obtain this constant oxygen reading, a half-dollar-sized electrode was placed on Janessa's skin with some type of sticky substance. It was crucial that the electrode be moved frequently, though, because intense heat forms under it. The amount of heat that collects under this electrode can result in a severe burn.

A premature baby's skin is very easily damaged, because it is so thin. Sadly, someone forgot to move this electrode during their shift one day. It must have been overlooked for quite some time, because the heat that built up underneath it caused a horrible burn on Janessa's tiny body. The result of this person's negligence is that there's a permanent burn scar in the exact shape of that round electrode. How tragic and how preventable!

Some days, I wasn't able to be at the hospital during the

morning. But, I constantly wanted to know how Janessa was doing when I wasn't there. At those times, I'd call the perinatal center at least once per shift to check on her progress. Many times during such calls, I received news that she had lost some weight or that her oxygen had to be increased or that she had stopped breathing, requiring resuscitation. I can vividly remember hanging up the phone at the end of those discouraging calls and crying. Within a few minutes, though, I would pick myself up and encourage myself. Some of those times, I would start singing, even though the report hadn't given me a reason to sing.

The medical profession could only base their reports on the physical symptoms they observed. They were giving me the facts as they saw them. Unfortunately, most people who receive negative reports camp in the middle of that negativity. So, if a situation looks bad to them, they expect the worst.

I understand that thinking. However, GOD is NOT visible to the natural eye. Yet, He is as real as you are. Because he IS so real, yet unseen, we can honestly say that visible things are not MORE real than God is. I had to make a decision as to whether I would believe the professionals' reports that were based solely on visible signs, or would I believe what God says in his word?

Here's a good example of what I mean. After Janessa had been on the respirator almost five weeks, she was still not able to be weaned from it. Each time they'd tried removing the breathing tube to place her under an oxygen hood, she went downhill fast. They would then have to reconnect her to the ventilator again. She seemed to be so dependent on the respirator they said she may never breathe on her own without assistance. That's what it LOOKED LIKE to them. But, THAT was subject to change.

In spite of these repeated failures, the very next day after the awful report, Janessa managed to pull the breathing tube out of her throat with her own tiny matchstick-sized fingers!

Unknown to the nurse on duty, the tube was laying barely inside Janessa's mouth. But, the oxygen reading was great.

When they discovered the dislodged breathing tube, they were shocked that Janessa was breathing on her own and maintaining such a good oxygen level. The tube was completely removed, and she was placed under an oxygen hood. From that day forward, she was NEVER on a ventilator again. But, just the day before, I had been told she would likely be on it forever.

Now that she was breathing on her own, she could be introduced to a baby bottle. At five weeks of age, she had never been fed with a bottle. She had received all of her nutrition through IVs or from the little bits of sugar water or breast milk placed into her stomach via a tube in her throat. A few times, she had been given a preemie baby-bottle nipple stuffed with cotton balls as a makeshift pacifier. This didn't happen very often, though. A nurse explained to me that some newborns who go this long without sucking are never able to do so properly. There was some concern that Janessa might have a problem in this regard.

Lo and behold, the attempts to feed her by bottle resulted in yet another negative report. It seems that Janessa did fine at taking the bottle, but something in her digestive system just did not work properly. Her formula intake by mouth was not matched by any bowel elimination. This was a real cause for alarm, and I was told that it could be an indication that she had developed a serious intestinal disease commonly associated with premature babies.

They attempted over and over again to feed her by mouth, but her intestinal tract was just unable to tolerate it properly. Each time she was fed, they would later insert a small tube down her throat and into her stomach to withdraw and measure whatever remained there from the feeding. This would tell them how much formula was being digested. It was so disheartening when the amount they withdrew each time was almost equal to the amount she had just ingested.

Their concern grew more and more as the days passed. I was told that this problem could be caused by an intestinal condition that frequently requires surgical removal of some sections of the intestines. They were preparing me for the worst. However, just a few days after I was told that she might need this surgery, her intestines suddenly started working perfectly! There was no physical explanation for why or how it happened. Her intestines just started working like they should. Thus, another negative report was totally reversed.

One after another, the situations that looked so hopeless were turned around. I received many bad reports that were based on visible signs and symptoms, and I've mentioned only a few of them here. One of the most important things I learned while walking through this ordeal is that I must NEVER be shaken by the way things look. Everything that can be seen is subject to change!

Chapter 9

Daily Medical Records

In order to accurately report the details of Janessa's birth and hospitalization, I purchased a copy of her medical records from the hospital where she was born. These next few chapters are devoted to giving some of the details recorded by doctors, nurses, and technicians in daily records.

The explanations of medical terms that you will see in parentheses were not in the hospital records. I have added these definitions for the reader in hopes of bringing clarity via a medical dictionary. The medical terms are in the hospital records, but I've added the definitions here.

Every line from each day's written notes will not be given. But, enough information from the three-month stay will be provided to give you a clear picture of what took place. For the first month, June, I list daily notes. For the remaining two months, I condense information. Please note that there is a nurse's daily chart referenced, and there's also a separate doctor's daily chart that is frequently mentioned, as well.

If anyone who's reading this is going through a similar situation or one that seems equally hard, I pray that this story becomes a beacon of hope for you. There truly was a light at the end of my tunnel, and it WAS NOT an oncoming train.

For those readers who are not detail-oriented, you may want to just skip this part entirely or mainly skim through it. However, for those readers who love details, this is for you!

Janessa's medical records begin with her admittance to the perinatal center at 9:45 PM on May 30, 1981, just 12 minutes after her birth.

<u>Day 1</u> - (May 30)

The "Special Care Nursery Admission Sheet" that was completed when Janessa arrived at the perinatal center documents her weight as 870 grams at birth, which converts to 30 ounces. Her length is listed as 35 centimeters, or barely over 13 inches. On the section of the sheet titled Respiratory Effort, the word "Absent" is marked, indicating she had no signs of breathing on her own. The form also shows she was placed on a Sechrist respirator / ventilator and was receiving 100% oxygen.

A second form completed the same night indicates that Janessa was born during the 26th week of my pregnancy. A full-term pregnancy is 38 - 40 weeks, making Janessa 12 - 14 weeks premature. This form lists her Apgar score as three at birth. After respiratory assistance, a second Apgar evaluation was done when she was five minutes old. The score had now increased to a six, solely due to the breathing help she was receiving.

This form notes that she was cyanotic (bluish-colored due to insufficient oxygen in the blood) and that she was in respiratory distress when the team of specialists received her at birth in the delivery room. She required continual bagging (a resuscitation method using an instrument that fits over the mouth and nose. It requires manually squeezing and releasing a flexible bulb to force air into the lungs.) Bagging was necessary until a tube could be inserted into her mouth and down into her trachea to connect her to a respirator. At 11 PM, her oxygen level on the ventilator was lowered from 100% to 85%. So, the air pumped into her lungs was a mixture of 85% oxygen & 15% room air.

The first day's record is two hours and 15 minutes long. Each day's record ends at midnight, and a new day begins.

<u>Day 2</u> - (May 31)

Just after midnight, an IV was started in Janessa's scalp. So, some hair had to be shaved from her head to create a sterile spot. Believe it or not, even though she was born so prematurely, she had quite a bit of light brown hair.

From midnight to 2 AM, the oxygen setting on her respirator was dropped to 75%, then to 60%, and finally to 27%. The nurse's report states that Janessa's color remained pink, and she showed no sign of distress from having the oxygen lowered. A couple of times it was observed that she exhibited spontaneous respiration, meaning that she tried to breathe a little on her own, although the respirator was mechanically pumping breaths into her at a rate of 40 times per minute.

There was some concern noted that Janessa had no urine output since arriving in the perinatal center. Between 9 PM and midnight, 24 hours after birth, there was only a small amount recorded. Urine output was measured by weighing the newborn disposable diaper on which she lay. They could determine a fairly accurate measurement of output, because they knew how much the diaper weighed dry.

It was extremely important for the doctors and nurses to know Janessa's blood gas levels regularly. That made it necessary for them to take blood from her frequently. The chart shows that blood was drawn six times on this day. It is no wonder that the chart also shows a notation saying, "baby irritable to touch." Barely 24 hours old, yet she had already begun to relate touch with pain.

The manner in which blood was drawn would cause anyone to cringe. Remember, everything on this baby was micro-miniature, so extreme diligence was required to hit a vein with the needle. Sometimes, the blood had to be drawn from an artery, but much of the time, it was drawn from her heel. Imagine what it was like for me to watch them stick Janessa's heel with a small razor-blade-type instrument, then grasp her heel in one hand and bend her foot straight up so that her toes touched the front of her leg. While holding that tiny foot in this awful position, the nurse would then squeeze downward with her thumb and forefinger, in essence milking blood from the bottom of Janessa's heel.

The first time I saw it, I was horrified. Janessa writhed in pain and cried, but no sound could escape, because the respirator tube in her throat kept her vocal cords from producing any sound. I cried with her as I watched.

The nurse who came on duty at 7 AM noted that Janessa appeared to be slightly jaundiced (yellowish color of the skin caused when an immature liver cannot properly process and remove old red blood cells as they are broken down). Additionally, at 2 PM, the IV in her head had infiltrated (fluid from the IV was leaking into the surrounding tissue instead of going into the vein). At 4:45, the IV was moved to her left arm. More needle sticks.

The doctor's report for today shows an elevated white blood cell count, indicating possible infection. An antibiotic was started through her IV.

Day 3 - (June 1)

At 3:30 AM, phototherapy was begun in order to control the jaundice. This involves placing a special intense light, a sort of black light, over the bed to help the baby's body rid itself (through the skin) of the broken down matter from the liver. A "Lone-Ranger-style" mask is placed over the eyes to prevent damage from the light.

By 5:20 AM, Janessa had only voided 5 CCs (around one teaspoon) of urine since her birth. Dr. K was notified due to the nurse's concern. The chart reads, "Unable to obtain enough urine for multistix" (test). The amount of fluid intake through the IV was increased for a fluid challenge test.

A notation says, "Skin very sensitive. What touches it leaves a mark. Abrasion on left side of chest present." Folks, this is the BURN that I mentioned earlier, caused by the oxygen sensor that was left too long in one place. Notice how this tragedy was not reported honestly in the nurse's note. This was NOT an "abrasion" caused by something touching the skin. It was a BURN, and the scar still remains TO THIS VERY DAY.

The nurse noted at 4 PM that she suctioned "thick, yellow, frothy, clear mucous from ET tube" (breathing tube). Then at 8:15 PM, the chart shows, "Color dusky. Breath sounds not audible in lungs. Extubated (removed breathing tube) and bagged (air manually forced in) with 80% oxygen for over 3 minutes. Reintubated (breathing tube reinserted). Ventilator setting at 30% oxygen."

<u>Day 4</u> - (June 2)

Starting at midnight, the nurse's chart reads, "Color pink and jaundiced. Active at intervals. Occasional respiratory effort noted. Remains NPO (nothing by mouth). Remains under phototherapy with mask covering eyes."

Dr. C is Janessa's attending physician for the month of June. An entry at 2 PM states, "Doctor C notified of increased blood pressure. EKG ordered" (test using small electrodes placed on the body to record the electrical activity of the heart). On the doctor's chart for this same time period, there is a notation stating, "EKG to check for hyperkalemia" (an abnormal increase of potassium that can profoundly affect the nervous system and heart, and when extreme, can be fatal).

The nurse's chart has a notation that says, "Dark discolored area on left side of chest." This is the BURN area that's NOT being called a burn in these records. An entry at 10 PM says blood was drawn directly from a left artery, and it took five minutes of constant pressure on the puncture site to stop the bleeding afterward.

Other items of concern shown on the doctor's report include, "Question as to whether patient is dehydrated. Urine output down. BUN level rising" (blood urea nitrogen - a compound from urine in the blood). Another notation says, "Ventilator dependent."

<u>Day 5</u> - (June 3)

Nurse's report - 2:30 PM - Remains under phototherapy with mask covering eyes. Plastic wrap covering body for body temperature.

3:30 PM - Phototherapy discontinued. 3:45 PM - Extubated (breathing tube out) and reintubated (tube reinserted).

A chest X-ray was ordered to check the position of the ET tube. For this procedure, a portable X-ray machine was brought to the bedside to eliminate moving the baby. The results showed, "ET tube is quite high in the neck and should be repositioned." This means Janessa was not fully getting the amount of oxygen she needed, since the tube wasn't down far enough into the lung area.

"4:00 PM - IV restarted in right foot. Baby extubated self during IV procedure. Placed under oxygen hood (a clear, hard plastic, shell-type hood that fills with oxygen and is placed over infant's head area) at 30% oxygen." Janessa had somehow dislodged her breathing tube. Apparently, her condition seemed to remain somewhat stable afterward, so it was decided that she would not be reconnected to the respirator. Instead, an oxygen hood was used. That meant Janessa was now totally on her own to breathe. I had grave concerns that she wasn't developed enough to handle that.

Sure enough, at 8:30 PM, a drastic change in Janessa's condition occurred. Within hours of the time that she was removed from the respirator and placed under the oxygen hood, her heart rate began to drop below acceptable levels. This condition is called bradycardia. Janessa NEVER had any trouble with it before now. The nurse's report states, "Brady 2 times. Heart rate in the 60s. Moderate to vigorous stimulation required." It took physical jolting, rousing, moving, and shaking by the nurse in both cases to cause Janessa's heart rate to return to normal.

The doctor on call that night notes that Janessa was having "some mild to moderate respiratory distress" and that her blood gases were "just adequate". He also states, "Baby had approximately 14 CCs of blood drawn so far in 24 hours and has not had any blood transfusion." He ordered a transfusion of 9 CCs immediately. Premature babies are not able to replenish their blood as fast as full-term babies can. So, even a small amount of blood loss can easily have a drastic effect on a preemie weighing less than two pounds.

Around 10 PM, this doctor ordered a blood test to determine the level of antibiotic in Janessa's bloodstream. Although no infection had shown up in the tests so far, an antibiotic was still being given.

Day 6 - (June 4)

Beginning at midnight, the nurse's chart says, "Color pink, pale, with slightly dusky undertones. Bradycardia with apnea (stopped breathing). Heart rate dropped to 50s. Required vigorous stimulation."

Since being removed from the respirator, Janessa was now experiencing episodes of apnea as well as bradycardia. The nurses noted ***12 instances in a 24-hour period!*** *Most of the notes show that it required moderate to vigorous stimulation to get her to start breathing again.*

Other concerns noted on the nurse's report include: "Head feels mushy. Urine output dropped. Skin broken down in several places on torso and extremities. IV started in left arm for 9 CCs of blood. Peripheral IV (main IV) restarted in right leg." Then a few hours later, another note reads, "IV restarted 2 times."

After the blood had been infused (over a 3 - 4 hour period), that IV was left intact in Janessa's tiny left hand but was not actively being used. The main IV was now in her left foot. SO MANY needle sticks must have been terribly painful for such a tiny little baby.

At 6 PM, the temperature control on Janessa's bed was lowered to 38 degrees Celsius (96.8 Fahrenheit) as the result of a nurse's notation at 4 PM that said Janessa's extremities were "warm to the touch." So, two hours later, the temperature was adjusted.

The doctor's report for the same 24-hour period reflects a rather troubling note: "Antibiotic dosage was 4 milligrams, 2 times more than needed. Decrease dose to 2 mg every 18 hours, and recheck levels in 2 days." WHAT?!! My tiny baby was receiving TWICE AS MUCH antibiotic as she should have, and a stand-in doctor discovered it!

Just to reiterate, the above revelation in the doctor's file about the overdosed antibiotic was put there by a "fill-in" perinatal center doctor, not Dr. C. Plus, Janessa was given her first blood transfusion EVER (to help replenish lost blood) by this STAND-IN doctor, NOT her own!

A lab report for this date gives the final results of testing done on cerebrospinal fluid taken from Janessa the day after her birth. Cerebrospinal fluid is the watery substance that surrounds the brain and spinal cord. This lab report shows that her fluid tested "negative" for streptococcus pneumoniae (the contributor to bacterial meningitis, (frequently fatal). Until I read the hospital report while doing research for this book, I was NEVER aware that Janessa EVER had a spinal tap done. NO ONE told me this!

<u>Day 7</u> - (June 5)
Here are some items on the nurse's report from midnight through 4 AM: "IV discontinued and restarted in right leg. Skin broken down in areas on torso and extremities. Scabs cracked and some minimal bleeding seen. Abdomen distended, but soft. Aspirated 10 CCs of air." This means air was drawn from Janessa's stomach via a tube placed down her throat. A small empty syringe was attached to the tube, and the plunger was slowly pulled outward.

At 4 AM, the IV was moved to her left leg. Later in the day, it was moved to her arm. She was voiding small amounts of urine. To again help control jaundice, phototherapy was restarted around 1 PM, after having been discontinued two days earlier. A blood transfusion of 8 CCs was given today.

Of great significance is a 2 PM note that reads, "Tolerated PO feeding (by mouth) of 2 CCs sterile H2o (water) without regurgitation." Up to this point, Janessa had received nothing by mouth. This was her seventh day of life and her first real feeding, even though it was just water through a tube down her throat.

While I was somewhat delighted to learn that my baby had been given something by mouth, I was seriously concerned about her ability to tolerate any new challenges when it seemed that she was deeply struggling in her ability to even breathe and maintain a normal heartbeat. The records for this day show that she experienced 14 episodes of bradycardia in a 24-hour period! Three of those times she stopped breathing entirely, and eight of those times she required vigorous stimulation to bring her heart rate back to normal.

The doctor's report states, "Significant brady requiring mild to moderate stimulation." However, the nurses who actually tended to Janessa had more accurately reported that it took "vigorous" stimulation. The doctor's report continues: "On theophylline (medicine that dilates airways and stimulates the heart and central nervous system). Will check levels tomorrow." Janessa has now been placed on medication in an attempt to help her breathe. Concerning the oxyhood, the doctor states, "Will wean slowly."

Dr. C further notes, "Respiratory distress syndrome - hyaline membrane disease" (a respiratory disease of newborns, especially premature babies, where a membrane composed of proteins and dead cells line the tiny air sacs in the lungs making it difficult or impossible to process oxygen. There is also a lack of pulmonary surfactant that allows air sacs to collapse. Surfactant is a fluid produced right before birth which keeps the lungs from filling with water. Surfactant is lacking, though, in babies born as early as Janessa.)

*A very disturbing statement at the bottom of the doctor's sheet reflects concern over the overdosed antibiotic in Janessa's blood. It says, "**At toxic levels;** dosage lowered and spaced to every 18 hours. Will await cultures & recheck levels."*

As I'm doing the research of Janessa's hospital records to write this book, I see several areas that merit extreme examination concerning the medical care Janessa has been getting during this terribly crucial stage of her little life.

(1) She's received OVERDOSES of an antibiotic that is now at a toxic level in her tiny bloodstream, (2) she frequently stops breathing and requires VIGOROUS stimulation to begin breathing again, (3) her heart rate is dropping VERY OFTEN, and (4) she is not receiving breathing assistance even though she is exhibiting major deterioration in her physical condition after being removed from the ventilator.

I had NO idea that she had been given overdoses of antibiotic. But, I do remember mentally questioning the decision to leave her struggling under the oxyhood instead of putting her back on the respirator.

Chapter 10

More Records

Day 8 - (June 6)
First, the doctor's report for this day: "Calories - inadequate. Pulmonary - 30% oxygen under hood. Retracting severely (chest and abdomen showing extreme rising and falling with each breath, indicating very labored and difficult breathing). Metabolic acidosis (too much acid in the body). Hematology report (blood) - iatrogenic anemia resolved." (Iatrogenic means caused by a doctor, medicine, or treatment.) This anemia notation indicates that Janessa had become anemic as the result of the medical treatment she had received, possibly the fact that too much blood had been drawn out of her body before she was given blood transfusions. The word "resolved" means that the condition has now been corrected, at least temporarily.

Another note on the chart says, "Physiologic jaundice - partially iatrogenic - intralipid." Again, this notation using the word iatrogenic indicates that Janessa's jaundice is partly caused by the medical treatment she's getting. Intralipid is explained on Day 12 notes.

Now to the nurse's report for the day: "Midnight: Color pink / jaundiced. Large amount of thick, white/yellow colored PO secretions (by mouth). Tolerated midnight and 2 AM gavage feedings (by tube) fairly well. No significant aspiration or regurgitation. 4 AM feeding held (not given). 2.5 CCs of aspirate obtained and discarded."

This means much of Janessa's earlier two feedings stayed in her stomach for several hours without being digested.

The residue was then withdrawn before 4 AM with a small syringe attached to the end of her feeding tube. Due to this problem, she was not given a 4 AM feed. The 6 AM feeding was given, though, and the chart shows that she had 3 CCs.

The next notation has been circled on the chart by the nurse. It states, "Multiple episodes of apnea and bradycardia. Heart rate drops into the 60s. Responds with vigorous stimulation and suctioning of thick PO secretions." Janessa had now been off the respirator and under an oxyhood for three days and was having MAJOR problems with her heart and her breathing.

After shift change, the next nurse notes the following: "8 AM - Color pale pink. IV in left knee. Apnea and bradycardia with heart rate in the 60s requiring vigorous stimulation. Increased oxygen rate to 50%. Required bagging for 5 minutes. Dr. C notified and is at bedside." Twenty minutes later, the chart reads, "Oxygen lowered to 30%." Then, one hour and ten minutes later: "Apnea and brady with heart rate in the 70s. Required moderate stimulation." On the next nurse's shift, Janessa suffered two more identical spells.

A radiology report for this date indicates an X-ray was made of Janessa's abdomen. The diagnosis reads, "Pneumatosis intestinalis in the left abdomen." (This condition consists of multiple thin-walled, gas-filled cysts in the intestines.) Oh no, something new on the list of physical attacks against her tiny body.

Day 9 - (June 7)

Day nine of Janessa's life! Doctor's chart lists "Problem 1" for this day as being "Inadequate nutrition. Weight down to 1 pound and 11 ounces." While it's perfectly normal for newborns to lose weight shortly after birth, this can be critical for a preemie who has no excess weight to spare. Dr. C also says Janessa will be given a full seven-day course of the antibiotic she's getting "due to maternal (mother's) fever at delivery." When I saw this in the chart, I was shocked. I was NEVER told that I had a fever before nor during delivery.

The activity and observations written on the nurse's chart for today show the high level of adversity presently facing Janessa. The notations at the start of the day's chart (midnight) read, "Color pale pink. Moderate thick white PO secretions. Skin remains dry and irritated in places. Betadine ointment (antiseptic) applied to ankles. Baby slightly more active than 24 hours ago - weak cry noted at times."

The next statement begins this day's documentation of her heart and breathing difficulties. It says, "Apnea with bradycardia 3 times during 8-hour shift." The chart then lists more episodes that ultimately total ***10 times during a 24-hour period*** *where Janessa's heart rate dropped, and she completely stopped breathing!*

On top of these problems, the main IV in Janessa's right hand infiltrated and had to be restarted in her scalp. It was so hard for me to look at her without crying when I saw an IV needle protruding from her head.

A notation at 6 PM states, "Color very pale. Brady 2 times with apnea. Lethargic. Notified Dr. C." The nurse was so concerned about Janessa's condition that she called for the doctor. A notation written an hour and a half later reads, "IV started in right arm for blood transfusion." Janessa was given 9 CCs of blood, but the nurse still shows concern about Janessa's condition at 9:30 PM. She writes, "Blood infusing. Color remains pale - ashen. Brady 2 times - heart rate in the 60s with apnea."

After the 11 PM shift change, a notation says: "Color pale pink and slightly mottled." Just before midnight, a major decision was made concerning Janessa's treatment. She was placed back on a respirator. Finally! after four days of constant downhill momentum, she's getting help.

The oxygen level on the respirator was set at 30%, and the rate of breaths per minute was set at 20. Fifteen minutes later, the rate was increased to 25. The nurse's note then reads,"Tolerated intubation well without distress. Color more pink - less mottled." Thank goodness Janessa was now going to get some much needed assistance with something that had exhausted her tiny reserve of energy for days - breathing!

<u>Day 10</u> - (June 8)
Only once on the nurse's chart for this day is there a reference to brady. That notation reads, "9 AM: Having periods of apnea, but heart rate isn't dropping; full ventilator control. Remains pink." Three other notations by nurses throughout the day indicate, "No apnea or bradycardia." What a relief, and what a drastic change from the previous four days spent struggling under an oxyhood!

The IVs in Janessa's head and right arm had infiltrated, so both of them were discontinued. The main IV was restarted in a different spot on her scalp. The record shows that she was pricked nine other times this day for various blood tests, sometimes in her heel, but other times in her arm to draw blood from an artery instead of a vein.

A nurse's note at 2 PM states, "Abdomen firm & distended. Gavage tube placed - 8 CCs of air and 2 CCs of clear mucous aspirated (drawn out). Abdomen less distended afterward. Babe quite active." At 4 PM, Janessa was once again placed under the bili light (phototherapy) for jaundice. This treatment had been an on-again /off-again procedure for days.

Early in the morning, a CT scan (Computed Tomography Scan using X-rays) was completed on Janessa's brain. The technician's report states, "(1) Brain density and pattern are normal, without evidence of mass effect, and (2) The ventricles (chambers of the brain) and sulci (furrows, grooves) are within normal range for a patient of this age." Well, this is certainly welcome news!

The nurses would sometimes add a small postscript on the chart showing that I had called. This day says that I called three times - 6:30 AM, 10:15 AM, and 2:45 PM. Since no calls from me were recorded for the evening or night hours, this was probably a day that I was at the hospital during that time.

Lastly, the doctor's report lists "metabolic acidosis" as one of the problems Janessa faces. The medical dictionary says this is a condition with too much acid in the body. It can be caused by severe dehydration and low blood volume.

Day 11 - (June 9)

Dr. C's report lists some of Janessa's problems. One is "Inadequate nutrition," so there's an order to "gavage feed" (by tube). Another note orders the antibiotic that Janessa had been given continuously since birth to be discontinued.

At midnight, the bili light (for jaundice) was turned off, but it was turned back on at 6 AM. Shortly after midnight, the nurse reported, "Color dusky. Mouth suctioned. Abdomen distended, but soft. Tube passed 5 CCs of air aspirate" (air was drawn from Janessa's stomach through a tube).

"1:15 AM - Baby extubated. 1:20 - Reintubated. Color improved after intubation. 1:30 - X-ray for ET placement (to see if the breathing tube is in the correct spot). 6 AM - No apnea or brady." The oxygen level on the respirator was dropped to 35% at 3:30 AM, but was increased to 40% shortly after noon. No apnea nor bradycardia was noted today, so it sure seems that placing Janessa back on the respirator was definitely the right thing to do.

A rather alarming notation was recorded at 10 AM. "Aspirated stomach of 1 CC of dark, coffee-ground-type mucous. Tested guiac positive (substance was tested and showed blood was present). Dr. C notified. Feedings held." Not only did Janessa's feeding not properly digest, but now the residue has blood in it.

At 8 PM, an IV was started in Janessa's right hand to begin infusing 10 CCs of blood. During one of the many transfusions that Janessa received, I talked with a nurse about the procedure. She explained that each bag of blood was used for transfusing as many as three babies, one at a time. I have no idea how much blood Janessa received while in the perinatal center, but this time frame was just before AIDS became publicly exposed. Donated blood was not being checked for the presence of AIDS.

Day 12 - (June 10)

A problem listed on the doctor's report says, "Mild metabolic alkalosis." This means that Janessa's condition has now turned from acidosis to alkalosis (an abnormal condition of too much alkaline in the body, resulting from excessive alkali intake or from excessive acid loss). This is the exact opposite of her former condition.

The report shows her weight is up to 1 pound, 14 ounces. I am sure that the nurse deducted the weight of the tongue depressor taped to Janessa's right hand and arm to keep her IV intact. Each day now, there is a note from the doctor with orders to begin weaning Janessa from the respirator. I had hoped that they would at least let her regain some strength before trying that again.

Another note reads, "Attempting to feed today. Sterile water feeds." This is the first attempt to feed Janessa after blood was discovered in her stomach yesterday.

One questionable notation on the chart says, "Remains on antibiotic." This note is very confusing to me, because it is in direct contradiction to yesterday's file that says the antibiotic was discontinued.

The nurse's chart reads, "Midnight - Head edematous (swollen due to excess fluid accumulation) and mushy. IV in scalp vein discontinued and restarted in right hand. Blood finished infusing earlier at 11:30. Color pink." A note is then written and circled. "Urine output down. Voided at 3:00. Urine concentrated and dark amber in color."

The evening nurse states, "Dependent edema (swelling)

noted in head. Abdomen appears slightly distended, but soft. IV infusing well in right ankle. Color pink. Infant active at intervals. 8 PM - Intralipids started. (Explanation follows.)

(Lipids are fatty substances that, along with proteins and carbohydrates, make up the three main parts of living cells. They also serve as a source of fuel for the body. Lipids are vital for sustaining life.) So, according to the nurse's note, Janessa is now getting lipids by IV. My questions is: Should she have been getting them before her twelfth day of life?

The last note for the day reads, "No apnea or bradycardia noted." That's two days in a row without any breathing or heart rate issues now that she's back on the respirator.

Day 13 - (June 11)
At midnight, the nurse's report shows, "Pink, active. IV is infusing well in right ankle with no redness or edema at site. Dependent edema to head." Then at 2 AM, "Infant became very dusky colored and heart rate dropped to low 100s. Suctioned a large amount of white secretion from ET tube. Infant pinked up quickly."

I consider the next statement to be monumental. "Tolerated well 4 CCs of donated breast milk by gavage tube with no regurgitation." For the very first time in her 13-day life, Janessa was given milk! The hospital maintains a supply of donated breast milk especially for the purpose of feeding critical babies. This gives these struggling infants the extra nutritional benefit that breast milk provides, and Janessa was now a bona fide beneficiary.

Unbelievable, this doctor decided at 9:50 AM to make a drastic change in her care. My tiny baby was removed from the respirator and placed on a machine called "Continuous Positive Airway Pressure" or CPAP for short. This technique aids breathing by maintaining a constant air pressure in the lungs and airway. It usually involves placing a snug-fitting mask over the nose and mouth. This machine doesn't help the infant take breaths, but merely keeps a mild constant pressure pushing air into the baby's airway.

Well, about four hours after Janessa was taken off the respirator, there was a report of "Bradycardia - heart rate of 93 with apnea. Recovered with mild stimulation." Then again at 2:40 PM, "Bradycardia into the 90s with two episodes of apnea. Dusky color. Recovered with mild stimulation."

A decision was made at 3 PM to place Janessa back on the respirator. The oxygen level was set at 35%, but only five breaths per minute were being delivered. Janessa was essentially doing most of the breathing on her own but was receiving just a little boost from the respirator. Near the end of the day's chart, it reads at 10 PM, "Color pink. Infant active at intervals. No apnea or bradycardia noted." She was proving that she obviously WAS NOT ready to be off the respirator yet.

The doctor's chart for this day reveals some serious concerns. One notation reads, "Possible sepsis" (a blood stream infection). Several lines follow: "New problem - possible NEC. Feedings held today. Abdominal X-ray showed questionable areas suspicious of pneumatosis (abnormal accumulation of gas). PO feedings (by mouth) held. Abdominal X-ray at 2 PM not diagnostic. A CBC ordered (complete blood count) with platelets (elements of blood that assist clotting) and several X-rays to evaluate."

NEC is necrotizing enterocolitis, an extremely serious condition. It can affect both the large and the small intestines. The word necrosis means death of living tissue. The cell death is caused by the progressive, destructive action of enzymes in the intestines. Premature babies have immature, fragile bowels that are very sensitive to changes in blood flow and infection. When Dr. K held that previous meeting with me, she had explained that NEC is a very common problem in preemies. It frequently results in surgical removal of portions of the intestines. Tragically, it often results in death.

Included here are two X-ray reports. The first concerns a chest X-ray and states, "ET tube (breathing tube) appears to be satisfactory. Mild alveolar atelectatic changes (partial collapse of lung) seen in the right lung. Aeration appears to be slightly worsening. Somewhat irregular and deflated loops of small bowel in the upper portion of the abdomen, suspicious for NEC. No free air can be identified."

The second report is from an X-ray of Janessa's abdomen at 2:25 PM: "Intestinal gas appears to be slightly increased. There is still deflated small bowel at the left upper quadrant of the abdomen. No definite pneumatosis can be identified."

<u>Day 14</u> - (June 12)
Around 2 AM, the nurse records, "Occasional periods of becoming dusky with heart rate dipping down, especially after any stimulation" (touch). Then at 6:30 - "Baby has rested quietly most of the night with no distress noted when there is no stimulation. Approximately 3 episodes of heart rate dropping into the 90s without apnea, all occurring when stimulated." Janessa was responding very adversely when touched. For her, touch meant pain. This breaks my heart.

The second nurse for the day notes at 7:30 AM: " Bradycardic. Secretions in ET tube. Suctioned tube, and heart rate began to increase. During episode, color was cyanotic" (blue). Blood was drawn at 9:40 from an artery to do a blood culture. At 10:30, a second IV was started for a blood transfusion. Only one notation during the evening hours showed an episode of bradycardia.

The blood drawn on this day for a culture will be observed by the lab for four days. The results on June 16 will show that Janessa's blood is positive for staphylococcus (a bacteria which is the main culprit in hospital-acquired infections, and which causes thousands of deaths each year). This infection is commonly called a staph infection. Now, it's a major threat to Janessa's welfare.

Two X-rays were done on her abdomen. The tech's report for the one completed at noon says, "(1) Gas-filled loops of small and large bowel are again noted, and (2) Bubbly-appearing radiolucency (permits X-rays to pass through) in the left mid-abdomen and some bubbly irregular lucency in the right side of the flank. Findings are still suspicious for necrotizing enterocolitis."

The second X-ray was taken at 8:14 PM, and the results were: "Gas is seen in large and small bowel loops. There are changes in the left abdomen suspicious for early pneumatosis intestinalis. Incidental note is made of changes in both lungs consistent with HMD" (hyaline membrane disease).

The last notation on the page says, "Impression: suspect early pneumatosis intestinalis (gas-filled cysts) in left abdomen." Needless to say, this is NOT a good report.

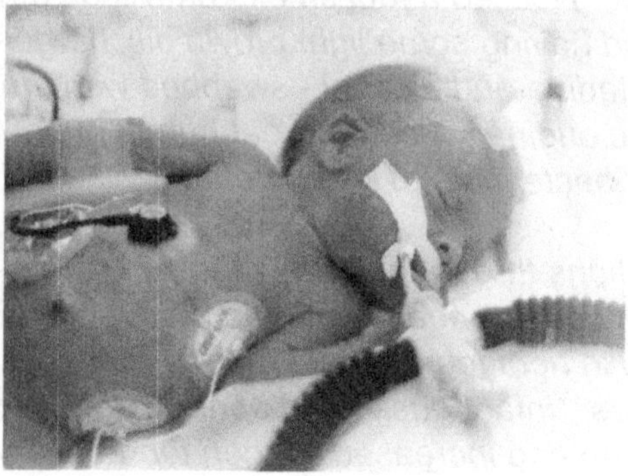

- almost 5 weeks old -
just days before coming off the respirator

Chapter 11

Records Continued

Day 15 - **(June 13)**
Nurse's report: "3:00 AM - Brady 3 times with heart rate dropping into the 70s. Color cyanotic (blue). Suctioned ET tube and received a moderate amount of white secretion. 6:00 AM - Awake, alert, and active with stimulation and at infrequent intervals. IV in right leg is infusing well. Brady with duskiness when suctioned."

After the 7 AM shift change, it reads, "Color pink with dusky under-tones. Active at times. Usually increased duskiness when touched. Noticed a foul smell - umbilicus (naval) reddened and having some light brown discharge - cleaned area with betadine and alcohol - swabbed with triple dye" (an antiseptic originally used to treat burns, but now used as a general bactericide to kill bacteria).

Further notations through the day read: "2:00 PM - Dusky off and on all day - apnea noted. No brady, however. IV discontinued in right leg and restarted in scalp." An entry at 6 PM states, "Infant dusky and apneic. Required vigorous stimulation and increased oxygen for recovery. Occasional shallow respiration."

Earlier in the afternoon at 2 PM, some of the secretions extracted from Janessa's breathing tube were sent to the lab for examination. The culture would be observed for two days and will reveal the presence of staphylococcus, just like her blood culture that was drawn the day before will eventually show. No one is aware of this yet, though.

The doctor's report lists concerns for this day: "Became acidotic with some CO2 (carbon dioxide) retention. Ordered increased rate to 15 (of respirator breaths per minute). Has apnea & brady episodes, frequent today. Patient gets angry and becomes dusky colored when touched. Blood gases have been good to bad. Frequent respiratory acidosis (is caused by excessive retention of carbon dioxide due to respiratory abnormality). 11 PM - oxygen raised to 40%. Repeat CBC (complete blood count) in AM."

<u>Day 16</u> - (June 14)

First, today's chart has a positive report! A chest and abdomen X-ray was completed at 8:30 AM. The tech's report states: "The lung fields appear better aerated than the last study. Moderate amount of bowel gas is present. No pneumatosis identified. Impression: Improved pulmonary ventilation. No diagnostic abnormalities in abdomen."

What a wonderful report! This is a welcome reversal of the previous assessment. Improved ventilation in the lungs, and no pneumatosis.

The report given by Janessa's nurses for this day required a page and a half instead of the usual one page. Starting at midnight: "Abdomen distended and soft. Inserted a tube into stomach - aspirated 7 CCs of air. Abdomen girth reduced by .5 centimeters (approximately 1/5 of an inch). Episodes of duskiness with heart rate dropping to low 100s three times. Increased the oxygen level and stimulated. Color pink now and heart rate increased to 130s - 150s. Dusky undertones to baby's color."

The notation written at 4:45 AM was very alarming for me to read when doing research for this book. I was NEVER told about this incident, which could have had VERY serious consequences for Janessa. The entry states, "Recalibrated oxygen analyzer and found it to be 14 points too high. Analyzer has been reading 42% oxygen, but infant was only receiving 28%. Analyzer now calibrated properly."

WHAT?!! A tiny baby has exhibited obvious signs of respiratory distress FOR DAYS - dusky and blue-colored. Episodes with no breathing at all. A dropping heart rate. Then, a notation in the records shows that her oxygen analyzer is faulty ... by a whopping ***14 points!***

Reading this type of disclosure in the hospital notes makes me realize even more that God was the one taking care of Janessa, not mere humans. Please remember also that during this time frame, Janessa was battling a staph infection that the doctor and the nurses know nothing about yet.

At 6 AM, another tube was inserted into her stomach. This time, 6 CCs of air were extracted. An hour later, another tube insertion removed 12 more CCs of air and 2 CCs of clear mucous from her stomach.

Several notations throughout the day make reference to her poor color. "Baby's color dusky. Brady 3 times requiring vigorous stimulation before 4:45 AM. Became very dusky with tactile stimulation (touch) and suctioning. Gets dusky when touched. Otherwise pink when quiet. Continues to have frequent periods of duskiness associated with shallow breathing or apnea. Apnea with bradycardia and duskiness requiring vigorous tactile stimulation for recovery. Infant becomes extremely cyanotic (blue) when touched."

Day 17 - (June 15)

A chest X-ray at 7:30 AM produced the following report from the physician who interpreted it. "(1) Diffuse pulmonary opacities are noted (widely distributed particles of some kind in the lungs reducing transmission of light and obstructing the view in the lungs). Exact etiology (cause and origin) of these changes is not known. The changes are not typical of hyaline membrane disease. (2) The heart is normal in size. (3) Endotracheal tube is well positioned. Impression: Diffuse pulmonary opacities of unknown etiology, probably not significantly changed since yesterday."

Janessa endured several horrific rounds of IV needles.

Around midnight, the IV in her right arm became swollen and was discontinued. It was restarted in her left arm. At noon, an IV was started in her scalp for a blood transfusion. Half an hour later, however, the IV in her left arm infiltrated, was removed, and a new one was started in her right hand.

"8:30 PM - Bradycardia with apnea and duskiness requiring vigorous stimulation and increased oxygen for recovery two times on this shift." It should be obvious to everyone that Janessa is not doing well at this time.

The doctor's chart shows, "Inadequate nutrition" along with a note stating, "Infection not a problem." This is an assumption on his part that will soon prove to be very wrong. When lab results return for the blood work and culture done days ago, it will show that Janessa has been battling a roaring staph infection for quite some time now!

A chart section concerning Janessa's respiratory function reads, "Continues to have bradycardia. Monitor registers an alarm, but no change noted in her physical appearance. Will get 12-hour apnea recording."

It is beyond me how this doctor could write that there is no change in Janessa's physical appearance with these episodes that set off the alarm on her monitor. That statement is in direct contradiction of the nurses who are clearly noting Janessa's poor coloring and the need for "vigorous" stimulation and "increased oxygen" to help her pull out of these episodes! It doesn't even sound like this doctor is talking about the same baby that the nurses are!

<u>Day 18</u> - (June 16)
On the doctor's chart, Dr. C wrote, "Weight - .98 kilograms (2 pounds and 2 ounces). On 45% oxygen. Possible sepsis (blood stream infection). On no antibiotics. Blood culture shows positive at 103 hours (on the 4th day) for cocci (staph bacteria). Will redraw blood culture and follow CBC." They've now gotten the results of the blood culture drawn FOUR DAYS AGO. It shows the staph infection that she

has had for at least four days with no medical treatment yet.

A new blood culture was done on this day, and two more follow-up blood cultures were done the next day. Amazingly, all of these cultures came back showing "No Growth." Janessa had not been given any antibiotic during this time period, yet the staph infection that had been detected in TWO separate cultures has now completely disappeared! TO GOD BE THE GLORY!

A chest and abdomen X-ray was taken at 7:30 AM. The results say: "(1) Diffuse densities in both lungs are again noted. These changes may be secondary to broncho-pulmonary dysplasia (a chronic lung disease in infants who have received mechanical respiratory support with high levels of oxygen in the first several weeks after birth), (2) There has been no change in the appearance of the lungs or heart size since previous study, and (3) Gas pattern in the abdomen is within normal variation." It seems there is now speculation that Janessa could be developing a lung disease caused by being on the respirator so long.

From midnight through 7 AM, the following notes appear on the nurse's chart. "Color pink at rest. ET secretions. Becomes dusky easily with any stimulation. Becomes bradycardic with heart rate in the 90s and dusky when suctioned.

Required bagging and oxygen at 60% for 2-3 minutes to recover from bradycardic episode. Aspirate that was removed (suctioned out) tested positive for blood. Infant active and fussy easily, especially when wet. Apnea and brady episodes 7-8 times with heart rate into the 60s and 70s. Required stimulation as above." Janessa is having a terrible time with her breathing and heart rate.

A notation at noon reads, "Dusky when stimulated." Then at 3:30 PM: "Remains pink at rest, but dusky upon stimulation." However, no episodes of bradycardia nor apnea are recorded from 8 AM through midnight. The respirator setting stayed at 45% oxygen with 30 breaths per minute.

On a second page for this date, the only item written is a small paragraph from the hospital social worker. It reads: **"Social Service Note:** *Conference with Dr. K. Parents appear to better understand seriousness of baby's condition." This note, along with the angry remarks Dr. K had made to me in our earlier meeting, gave me the impression that they mistook my calm assurance to be a lack of understanding just how critical Janessa's situation really was.*

Day 19 - (June 17)

Nurse's report: "Midnight to 7 AM - Tolerates stimulation poorly, especially being suctioned. Reacts with duskiness and heart rate dropping to 100. Responds well when bagged briefly and suctioned for mucous plugs. No bradycardia or apnea other than with suctioning."

"10:45 AM - IV started in left arm for blood transfusion." When the blood had finished transfusing, the nurse transferred Janessa's regular IV tubing over to the needle already in place from the transfusion. However, that IV started leaking around 6 PM, so it was discontinued and restarted in Janessa's scalp once again. Many of the pictures I have of Janessa from her time here in the perinatal center show an IV in her head.

Further notations on the chart read, "Blood cultures drawn from right radial and temporal. Pressure to sites for 5 minutes to stop bleeding. No hematomas (blood clots) or seepage at sites." Half an hour later, it reads, "Dr. C notified of arterial blood gas results."

No apnea nor bradycardia was noted on any other shift after the one instance when Janessa was being suctioned before 7 AM. Her respirator's oxygen level was lowered through the day from 45% to 40%. In addition, the number of breaths provided was dropped from 30 per minute to 25.

Dr. C's report states: "Ventilator dependent. Chest X-ray showed diffuse pulmonary opacities not suggestive of hyaline membrane disease. Infant getting transfused. Iatrogenic anemia (anemia caused by medical treatment). Rule out sepsis. Will get ET tube cultures. On no antibiotics at this time."

Day 20 - (June 18)

Well, this day started out with a bang! Shortly before 1 AM, Janessa somehow managed to extubate herself, so her breathing tube had to be reinserted by a respiratory tech. A chest X-ray was ordered to check the position of the tube. At 4:10 AM, Janessa again extubated her breathing tube, which was promptly reinserted. Another chest X-ray was done to check the tube position this time. Then, at 5:20 AM, Janessa unbelievably dislodged her breathing tube again! That's THREE TIMES in only four hours! Of course, it was immediately reinserted.

Here's what the nurse's report says after the third time: "Extubated and reintubated 3 times. Tolerated it well without significant distress. Babe is able to manipulate ET tube with her tongue easily, so tube was taped securely after the third reintubation." Janessa was making it perfectly clear that she wanted that tube OUT of her mouth.

The X-ray report for today reads: "(1) Diffuse pulmonary densities are again noted. There is an interesting linear lucency (bright, shining lines) coursing vertically just to the right of the superior mediastinum (the space between the lungs). An early pneumomediastinum (loose, free air in the space between the lungs where it does not belong) cannot be excluded. (This condition can require surgery to remove the air via a chest tube.) Pulmonary opacities are not changed. (2) The heart is normal. (3) The endotracheal tube (ET) is well positioned. (4) Abdomen is within normal limits."

So, there is now the threat of another serious condition - loose air in her chest. This information is another one of the findings that I formerly DID NOT know. There seems to be a mountain of heretofore unknown information that I'm discovering as I read her medical records in preparation for writing this book.

Day 21 - (June 19)
The nurse's report shows four instances of drawing blood and one chest X-ray taken during this 24-hour period. The IV in Janessa's left arm infiltrated at 3 AM and had to be restarted. Guess where? Her scalp!

At 10:20 AM, an IV was also started in her right ankle. The IV needle in her scalp was left intact, but was capped off with a heparin lock. Heparin is a liquid substance that prevents blood from clotting. This procedure leaves the needle inserted in the skin and allows IV tubing to be reconnected to the needle when needed. Later at 4 PM, an IV of intralipids (fats) was connected at this site.

A couple of notations make reference to the appearance of Janessa's stomach. "Abdomen slightly more distended, but still soft," Then, "Abdomen distended with visible bowl loops, but is soft." One nurse mentions a slight diaper rash. "Placed infant on her abdomen, cleaned area with Ivory, and left open to air. Rash more faint this afternoon."

Following this report is a very comforting note for a mother to read: "Infant sucks on ET tube and on pacifier." One of the nurses had created a make-shift pacifier by using a preemie-sized baby bottle nipple stuffed with a cotton ball. Janessa must have found this VERY soothing.

Two notations about problems: "4 PM - 1 CC aspirated from stomach before feeding. Dr. C notified. Feeding held per order. 8 PM - 0.5 CCs aspirated from stomach before feeding. Dr. N notified - ordered NPO" (nothing by mouth). These instances are very disappointing, since they indicate that the digestive tract was not properly functioning.

No apnea nor bradycardia is noted through the whole day, but a 10 PM entry reads, "Infant becomes dusky and skin oxygen level drops when disturbed." Janessa is sending a clear message: "DO NOT TOUCH ME!" Sadly, touch means pain for her.

The doctor's chart lists Janessa's weight as 2 pounds and 4 ounces now. It also states that she is once more suffering from iatrogenic anemia, probably caused by the loss of so much blood for so many tests. So, Dr. C has written an order for a blood transfusion in the morning. The chart does finish with an uplifting note for this day, though. "No evidence of infection."

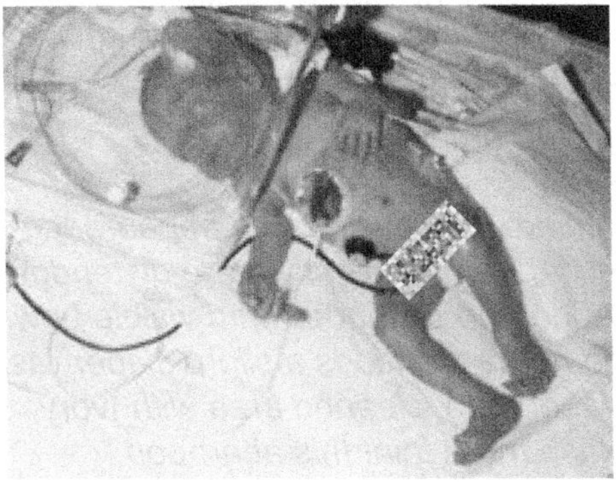

- 5 weeks old -
under an oxyhood

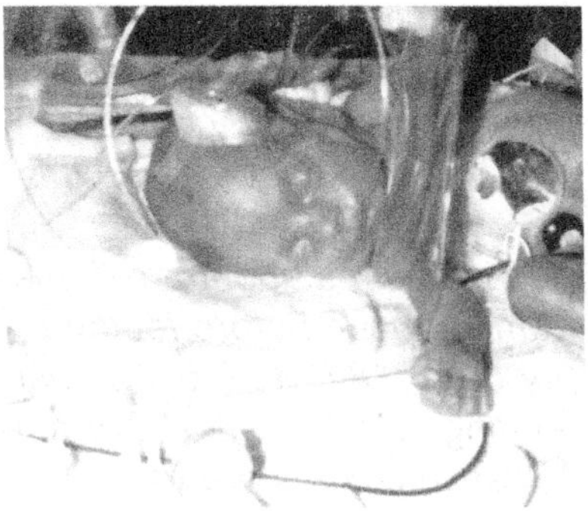

- 5 weeks old -
just after coming off respirator

Chapter 12

Daily Details Concluded

<u>Day 22</u> - (June 20)
By this time, I had begun to notice a trend. It became apparent to me that the apnea and bradycardia episodes increased dramatically when Janessa needed a blood transfusion. So, I started asking about her blood levels immediately when these spells began. My consensus was that she would be far better off to be given a blood transfusion right away when needed, rather than be forced to suffer through hours or days of breathing difficulties and heart rate drops first.

The doctor's report from yesterday indicates that a blood transfusion was ordered for this morning, but according to the nurse's report, blood wasn't started until after 4 PM. The effect that this delay had on Janessa seems to correlate exactly with my suspicions.

Nurse's notes follow: "Midnight to 7 AM - Duskiness with apnea and brady. Heart rate in the 90s for 3 - 4 minutes. Required moderate tactile stimulation and bagging briefly to recover. One other episode of brady with heart rate in the 90s. Responded with moderate tactile stimulation. No bagging required."

"7 AM to 3 PM - Periodic dusky episodes with skin oxygen level dropping. ***FIVE EPISODES*** *of heart rate dropping into the 70s and 80s, requiring mild to moderate tactile stimulation for recovery."*

The evening nurse also had her hands full as evidenced by

the numerous notes she wrote:
"3:30 PM - Skin oxygen level at ***17!*** *Cyanotic. Bagged with 35% oxygen for 2 minutes. Baby pinked up.*
8 PM - Skin oxygen level ***18!*** *Bagged for 10 minutes with 60% oxygen. Baby pinked.*
10 PM - Skin oxygen level ***21!*** *Suctioned small amount of liquid from ET tube. Bagged with 60% oxygen over 2 minutes. Pinked.*
10:45 PM - Baby doesn't tolerate suctioning well; yet needs suctioning often. No further bradycardia. Skin level is presently at ***47.****" Folks, dangerously low skin oxygen levels!*

An interesting note shows that I was at the hospital with Janessa at 9:30 PM. This means that I was there during the period when she was frequently requiring heroic efforts to revive her. Reading this note brings back vivid memories of the times when fear would try to grip me. Seeing her tremendous struggle to survive during those instances seriously impacted me. Each time I witnessed her near-death episodes, fear would try to tell me that she wouldn't be able to make it this time.

As mentioned earlier, the blood transfusion was started at 4:20 PM and was completed three hours later at 7:30. The IV in her scalp had infiltrated in the early morning hours and was restarted in another spot on her scalp. At 3:40 PM, an IV for intralipids was started in Janessa's left hand, but was then temporarily capped off with a heparin lock until the blood transfusion was completed at 7:30. At 8 PM, intralipids were restarted.

A chest and abdomen X-ray was done on this day. Only two days earlier, an X-ray had revealed abnormal linear lucencies (shiny lines) in Janessa's chest area. But today's X-ray showed that the problem had completely reversed. The report states, "I do not identify a pneumomediastinum." I can gladly say as her mother, "Thank you, God!" The note further shows, "Bowel gas pattern is within normal limits. No free air or portal vein gas is seen."

Day 23 - **(June 21)**

Because of the traumatic distress Janessa experienced during my hospital visit last evening, I phoned three times during this day to check on her progress. Once was around midnight, then at 8:50 AM, and again at 2 PM. According to the nurse's report, I was there at the hospital with Janessa at 9 PM.

It is important to note that I was rarely permitted to hold Janessa, because she was hooked to the respirator and IVs. During most of my hospital visits, I was only able to touch and gently talk to her. Amazingly, she didn't respond negatively to my touch. I spoke to her softly while doing so. Most likely, my familiar voice was a comfort to her, so she did not recoil and stop breathing like she did with the nurses.

This day turned out to be a much better day for Janessa than the day before had been. Only one entry reports any breathing or heart rate problems. So, it looks like the blood transfusion was a tremendous help, exactly as I expected it would be.

In reviewing the doctor's notes to write this book, I came across another interesting find. I discovered that the doctor didn't put any notes in Janessa's chart for this date. The page which should contain June 20 and June 21 skips the 21st altogether. It lists June 20 and June 22.

Day 24 - **(June 22)**

Around midnight, Janessa dislodged her breathing tube and required reintubation by a respiratory technician. Later, a second tube was temporarily inserted down her throat and into her abdomen. Through means of this additional tube, a large amount of air was drawn out, along with a scant amount of a yellow-green secretion. A 6:30 AM note says, "Active at intervals. Skin oxygen level drops drastically with agitation when disturbed. Some duskiness with crying. No apnea or bradycardia." As the day wore on, however, the battle with apnea and brady increased.

*"11:40 AM - Brady. Heart rate into the 80s and 90s with duskiness. Mild stimulation required. 2 PM- No further brady, but dusky episodes at intervals. Lowered tube into abdomen. 10 CCs of air with 1 CC of light brown mucous aspirated." Fifteen minutes later, a notation says: "Dusky spell without brady. Skin oxygen level dropped to **10!** Bagged for very short interval. Pinked up without problems."*

*At 4 PM, the nurse wrote, "Color pale pink." Then at 6 PM, "Bradycardia. Heart rate into the 80s. Dusky with poor perfusion (blood flow). Required bagging with 100% oxygen for **30 minutes!** Dr. C notified. Approximately 6 episodes of bradycardia requiring bagging between 6 PM and 7 PM."*

*The chart says that I was at the hospital at 8 PM. This means I was faced with yet another horrible day of awful episodes and reports. Janessa had required **30 minutes of bagging with 100% oxygen** to pull out of a potentially deadly tailspin. Believe me, if it had not been for the deep-seated, internal peace that God had given me, I would've completely broken down on a day like this.*

<u>Day 25</u> - (June 23)

Doctor's chart shows Janessa's weight as 2 pounds and 7 ounces. Another notation mentions respiratory acidosis again, and it further states that an increased oxygen rate does not seem to alleviate it. The final note reads, "Plan to CAT scan at earliest opportunity to rule out IVH" (inter ventricular hemorrhage - a blood hemorrhage in the brain).

Another day of multiple needle sticks for Janessa is shown on this report. Six times today. The notes again reveal how very concerned I was about Janessa's condition. This chart shows that I made a phone call around midnight in addition to another two calls between 7 AM and 3 PM. It is further recorded that I was back at the hospital by 6 PM.

The report also reads, "Midnight - Color pink and pale with occasional episodes of duskiness. Active when disturbed. 2 AM - Brady. Heart rate in the 90s. Skin oxygen level *dropped to **15!** Bagged for 2 - 3 minutes. Improved immediately." At 6 AM, Janessa was placed on her abdomen, which was very rarely done.*

"2 PM - Dependent edema (swelling) of head noted from previous IVs. Scalp IV discontinued. Restarted in scalp again. Apnea with brady. Heart rate in the 70s. Mild stimulation required. Duskiness." A further notation reads, "At intervals today, infant was dusky without brady. Required no stimulation to pink up. Active at intervals. Sleeping most of the time."

*The 3-to-11 nurse writes during her shift, "At times, turns dusky color and skin oxygen level drops. Recovers spontaneously. 7:40 PM - Skin oxygen level dropped to **10!** Dusky color. Bagged for 1 minute with 90% oxygen. Pink color returned and skin oxygen level measured 80%. At 8 PM, aspirated 3 CCs of white colored aspirate prior to attempting feeding by mouth. Dr. notified. Feeding held. Doctor ordered nothing to be given by mouth." The last notation for the day reads: "Color pink with skin oxygen level at 68. Baby active. No bradycardia this 8 hours."*

Day 26 - (June 24)

*Nurse's report: "Midnight to 7 AM - Color pink. Abdomen slightly distended, but soft. Dusky episodes 2 times without heart rate drop. Skin oxygen dropped to **20.** Recovered spontaneously when left undisturbed. No other distress."*

Note on the doctor's chart states, "Inadequate nutrition. Will feed today." The nurse's notes reflect the order: "Began feeds by mouth again at noon. 2 CCs of white mucous aspirated and discarded after shown to Dr. C. Gave 2 CCs of donated half-strength breast milk by tube. Scant amount of aspirate at 2 PM." Well, it seems that Janessa tolerated the milk better at this feeding.

*But, things would change at 8 PM. "1 CC of aspirate approximately 10 minutes after feeding. Color very dusky with heart rate dropping to the 90s. Skin oxygen reading **8!***

Bagged with 45% oxygen 5 minutes. Color improved."
10 PM - "2 CCs of green aspirate. Dr. C notified. Ordered nothing by mouth. 5 minutes after tube put down baby's throat into stomach to remove the aspirate, baby experienced bradycardia with heart rate into the 90s and dusky. Bagged for 3 minutes with 45% oxygen. Color improved after bagging."

<u>Day 27</u> - (June 25)

The first note on the doctor's chart reads, "Attempting to feed 2 CCs of half-strength breast milk every 2 hours without success." A notation concerning Janessa's lungs says, "Bronchopulmonary dysplasia due to prolonged mechanical ventilation." Additionally, a note regarding her heart reads, "No heart murmur has ever been heard."

Nurse's report expresses further concern about Janessa's tendency to turn a dusky color frequently. "Midnight: Babe became very dusky when weighed. Respiratory technician bagged, and skin color improved. ET tube secretions were thick and a copious amount (abundant). 2 AM: Babe opening eyes. Active intervals. Becomes dusky when attended / irritated!" Each nurse noted similar symptoms on this day.

The events mentioned next obviously contributed to the agitation Janessa experienced. She would tense and hold her breath when touched. No wonder!

"1 AM - Tube inserted into stomach through mouth. More than 20 CCs of air aspirated. 5:10 AM - Babe extubated self when turning head. Reintubated by respiratory technician. 5:25 AM - Chest X-ray to check ET tube placement. 6 AM - IV infiltrated. Restarted in left foot. Intralipids continue to infuse well into IV in left hand. Between 6 AM and 2 PM, IV changed to left lower scalp.

8 AM: Babe taken for CAT scan. 10 PM: 1.5 CCs aspirated from stomach. Dr. C notified. Feeding held. Scalp vein IV site edematous (swollen). Discontinued. Restarted in right hand." Five other instances of blood drawn for various tests are recorded for this day. Lastly, another treatment requiring touch: "10 PM - Glycerin suppository given."

I have saved the most encouraging information of the day for now. The radiologist's report of today's CAT scan gives some wonderful, welcome news. It reads, "Findings: The previous scan showed evidences of petechial identified hemorrhage (reddish spot containing blood) in the area of the caudate nuclei (section of the brain partially responsible for body movement and coordination) with subependymal hemorrhage (blood leaking under the membrane lining of the brain). But the current study (today's scan) shows a resolution of those areas of hemorrhage" (gone, resolved).

HALLELUJAH!! *The pools of blood previously found in Janessa's brain on the earlier CAT scan are gone now! No sign of them! Those pools of blood could have caused, or been a sign of, mental retardation. But, not anymore. They are GONE!*

<u>Day 28</u> - (June 26)

According to today's doctor's report, Janessa's nutrition continues to be a major concern. "Started 2 CCs of D5W (sugar water) every 2 hours by mouth today. Tolerated poorly, with scant to 1 CC of aspirate." Concerning her respiratory condition, the chart says, "Ventilator dependent for 28 days. Settings essentially unchanged. Has periods where she gets extremely dusky when stimulated or without stimulation. Question as to whether she is shunting" (abnormally diverting blood from its normal course).

Apparently, they have been unable to discern or explain what is causing the extreme duskiness that she frequently experiences. No obvious signs of organ abnormality. "No murmur. No cardiomegaly (enlarged heart) shown on chest X-ray. No palpable hepatomegaly" (no enlarged liver can be felt).

The nurse's chart begins with what might seem an insignificant notation at 3 AM - "Turned to left side." While this may not be earth-shaking news, remember that she has been entirely on her back for 28 days, except for a few brief moments on her abdomen.

No apnea nor bradycardia are noted for this 24-hour period. All of the three nurses, though, refer to the dusky episodes that Janessa continues to experience. The notation at 4 PM does give an upbeat report, however. "Tolerated 2 CCs of D5W by tube every 2 hours without significant aspirate or regurgitation." Wonder if there is any correlation between her improved digestion and being placed on her left side?

Day 29 - (June 27)

Janessa's weight is listed on the doctor's report as 2 pounds, 12 ounces. The nurse's report shows that blood was drawn four times this day for tests. The scalp IV did well all day. At noon, a second IV was started in Janessa's left foot for a blood transfusion. The respirator setting of 35% oxygen remained constant, but around 3 PM, the number of breaths per minute was increased from 25 to 30.

Very early in the morning, the nurse noticed that Janessa's body seemed to be holding too much fluid. Notation says, "Pitting edema (swelling that includes indentions in the swollen area) noted in lower extremities. Some dependent scalp edema noted. Eyes slightly puffy." According to later notes at 1:15 PM, the doctor must have ordered medicine to reduce the swelling. Report says, "Breath sounds were coarse earlier today, but are clear since Lasix was given." (Lasix is a diuretic that increases urine output to rid excess fluid from the body.)

A note at 7:35 AM indicates a small sample of tissue was taken from the remaining portion of umbilical cord that was still attached to Janessa's body. It was sent to the lab for a culture to test for bacteria. This lab report would be completed the next day.

The usual occurrences of duskiness continue. "Gets dusky when stimulated. Remains pink on current ventilator settings with periodic episodes of duskiness. Is dusky when disturbed." On a positive note, though, the feedings of sugar water are more successful than earlier, plus no cases of apnea nor bradycardia are reported.

Another bright spot among the various reports for this day is the radiologist's interpretation of Janessa's chest X-ray from 8:15 AM. It reads, "Considerable improvement in the right lung since yesterday. Impression: Re-expansion of the right lung." PRAISE GOD!! Janessa's right lung has now started to function properly!

<u>Day 30</u> - (June 28)
Just on the heels of the good news from yesterday about the lung, some serious concerns are documented on this day's report. Since this was a Sunday, another doctor was "on call" instead of Dr. C. This doctor, Dr. N, records these distressing facts: "I was called at 6 AM since the patient required constant bagging to maintain oxygenation. High pressures were required or bagging to move chest wall. Abdomen girth stable, but distended. Extremities (arms & legs) marked by pitting edema. Chest X-ray shows worsening of BPD (bronchopulmonary dysplasia - lung disease caused by respirator.) Ventilator settings altered until skin oxygen monitor was stable at around 60. Required ventilator settings of 70% oxygen at 40 breaths per minute."

Wow! This is indeed a step in the wrong direction. It is now taking much more oxygen to saturate Janessa's tiny body.

<u>Day 31</u> - (June 29)
She was given a blood transfusion at 8:30 this morning. Her chart shows she was stuck with needles ***10 times*** *to draw blood for testing blood gases. No wonder she needs to be given a transfusion so often. It is noted that she was very dusky, irritable, and crying earlier around 5 AM, plus she required bagging for 5 minutes. After she received the blood transfusion, though, she had no more duskiness on this day. When I look back on the entire month of records as I'm doing research to write this book, I often find myself*

extremely dismayed that this doctor allowed her to drop to such lows before he would give her much-needed blood.

End of the First Month

At the end of June, Janessa received a new doctor. The policy in the unit was to assign each doctor a set of critical babies to attend for one full month. At the end of the month, each doctor was rotated to a different set of babies. During the month, however, each doctor might have gained more babies as new ones were brought into the perinatal center. A rotating system was used to assign any new arrivals. Additionally, some doctors might have lost a few babies through an infant's dismissal from the hospital or from it passing away.

As each doctor finished the month of care for his or her set of babies, it was procedure for the doctor to write a detailed "Off Service Note" recounting each individual baby's history. I'll close out this chapter with a synopsis of the four-page dissertation written by Dr. C at the end of Janessa's first full month of life.

OFF SERVICE NOTE:

"Problem - Nutrition: Currently on parenteral nutrition (nourishment given other than through the intestines; such as by IV). Have attempted multiple times through the month to feed this child PO (by mouth). She has not tolerated breast milk, D5W, or sterile H2O. Gets abdomen distention. Calories per day are inadequate with protein and intralipid. You must re-attempt to feed at earliest opportunity or she could develop retention jaundice due to prolonged TPN" (total parenteral nutrition)."

"Problem - Ventilator dependent at present time. Initially, attempts were made to wean. It was felt that she had chronic pulmonary insufficiency of prematurity and that she periodically shunts. On June 1, ventilator settings were 27% oxygen at a rate of 10 breaths per minute with a pressure of 12. She was weaned to a hood June 3 at 30% oxygen. Made attempts to wean her to room air. On the night of

June 7, she deteriorated, and by June 8, she was back on the ventilator with settings of 30% oxygen, 25 breaths per minute, and a pressure of 16. She is currently on 35%, 25 breaths, pressure 18.

On June 28, she deteriorated around 6 AM and required constant bagging. Her ventilator was increased to 70% oxygen, a rate of 40 breaths, pressure 24. Since then, she has been weaned down. A series of chest X-rays show as consistent with bronchopulmonary dysplasia. She will be very difficult to wean."

"Cardiac status: I have never detected a murmur, and there has never been any suggestion of congestive failure or cardiomegaly (enlargement of the heart)."

"Problem - latrogenic anemia: She has sustained multiple episodes requiring transfusion and to date has been transfused 11 times. She is O positive. Donor blood - O positive and negative."

"Problem - Sepsis (toxic condition from bacteria) : The initial blood culture on admission was negative. Then, on June 12, a blood culture grew staphylococcus epidermidis. Repeat cultures were negative. A full septic work-up was done on admit and was negative.

Because mother was fevered at delivery, we continued ampicillin and gentamicin (antibiotics) for a full 7 days from delivery. On June 27, a cord culture (umbilical cord) grew Klebsiella (a bacteria that can cause pneumonia, urinary tract infections, etc.) and Citrobacter Freundii (bacteria some-times found in blood, urine, and throat swabs). This has not been treated. No antibiotics at present. Blood cultures were drawn June 29 and are pending."

"Problem - Apnea / Bradycardia: Has episodes of brady with heart rate dropping to the 70s, sometimes requiring vigorous bagging. On Aminophyllin. No 12-hour recording has been done."

"*Problem* - Central Nervous System: CAT scan of June 25 showed resolution of small subependymal hemorrhage and slightly more ventricular dilation than previously. Certainly a bleed could account for her apnea / brady. A scan was done June 30 and results are pending. Scan periodically as needed."

"The parents do not really comprehend that this infant has a long, long way to go.
Good Luck!
Dr. C "

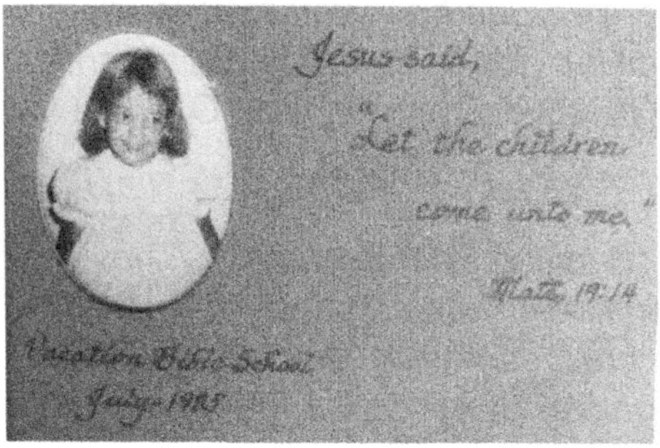
Jesus said,
"Let the children
come unto me,"
Matt. 19:14
Vacation Bible School
July - 1985

Janessa - age 4
Vacation Bible School

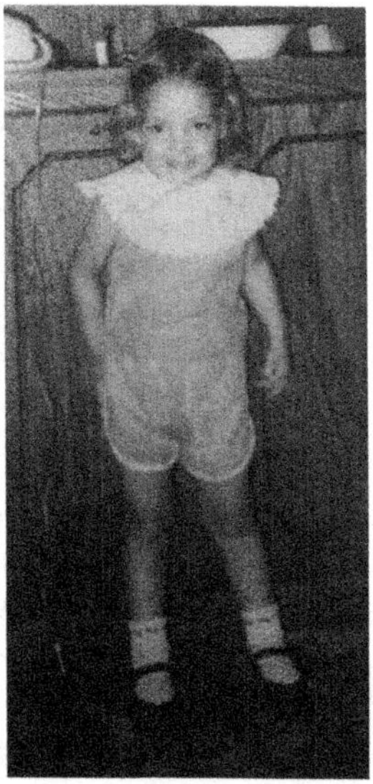

Janessa - age 3

- Oops! It looks like Dr. C forgot to mention that he gave Janessa overdoses of antibiotic to the point that she had toxic levels in her bloodstream.

Chapter 13

July & August

Dr. Cav (I'll call him) took over Janessa's case at the end of June. Under his care, the month of July would prove to be a time of major forward momentum in Janessa's life. One of the first things he did upon assuming her care was to write a standing order for her to receive a blood transfusion if her hemoglobin level dropped below 12. Formerly, she had not been transfused unless her hemoglobin level fell below 11.5. Often, her reading had gone well below that mark before she received any blood.

A few days after Dr. Cav's introduction, a dramatic change took place during the evening shift of July 3. Around 6 PM, Janessa extubated herself by somehow pulling the breathing tube out of her throat. When her nurse discovered the situation, Janessa's skin oxygen level was amazingly good, to the surprise of everyone. So, Dr. Cav decided to put Janessa under an oxygen hood with 35% oxygen instead of putting her back on the ventilator.

Mind you, this was within mere days of the first doctor's written dissertation in which he forewarned Dr. Cav that Janessa would be "very difficult to wean." Famous last words, Dr. C. Famous last words, indeed!

During the month of July, the setting for the oxyhood fluctuated from 35% down to 24%, then back up a bit as they tried to wean her to room air. She would often get dusky colored when they tried lowering her oxygen. One time, Dr. Cav wrote, "Patient yo-yo's from 24% to 28%."

Janessa continued to have some apnea and brady while under the hood. On July 18, a spinal tap was done, apparently to check for the presence of any disease that could be causing these episodes. The doctor's report says the spinal tap was bloody, so Janessa was started on antibiotics.

It is noted that Janessa sometimes experienced brady when the feeding tube was inserted down her throat or when it was withdrawn after a feeding. Additionally, for the first half of the month, she continued to have some problems fully digesting her formula each time. But on July 20, Dr. Cav ordered her feedings to be given every three hours instead of every two. This would allow more time for food to digest. According to the nurse's record, this theory on the doctor's part proved to be correct. From that time forward, Janessa began tolerating the feedings much better and had less aspirate and less regurgitation.

On July 18, she weighed 3 pounds and 6 ounces, almost double her birth weight. The nutrition IVs were halted on July 24. She was finally handling the gavage feedings (by tube) so well that she no longer needed a main IV. Only when she needed blood would they start an IV now.

The few Social Services notes in the records have always said things like the one that appears on July 24. It reads, "Family is under much stress and having some problems coping." These comments were likely prompted by the calmness that I continued to exhibit throughout this whole, long ordeal. Apparently, my peaceful demeanor was being interpreted as meaning that I had problems coping. (I am laughing on the inside as I type this.)

Interestingly, one week later on July 31, the same social worker who penned those words suddenly did a flip-flop! The things she wrote on the final day of July sound like she is talking about an entirely different family. Here's what she said, ***"Family situation remains stable. Parents remain encouraged about baby's condition."***

WHAT??!! That is NOT what she was saying just one week earlier! This is quite a change. Hmmm - maybe this social worker figured that she'd better catch up to the major progress Janessa was making, instead of trying to paint an awful, incorrect picture of gloom and doom.

On this same day, July 31, it was decided to let Janessa start feeding from a bottle. A small tube of flowing oxygen was held to her nose while she sucked on the bottle. She did amazingly well, but had to stop frequently to rest. It was a wonderful sight to behold! She did get some dusky undertones around her eyes and mouth from working so hard, but she pinked up afterward when she was returned to the oxygen hood.

At the end of July, Dr. Cav wrote a two-and-a-half page "Off Service Note" as he prepared to hand Janessa over to another doctor for the month of August. He did make a mistake in this report that I think is worthy of mentioning.

He starts by giving Janessa's birth history including the date, birth weight, and such. He then says, "Patient was born in a small outlying town and was transported to the perinatal center." Ummm, no. That is totally wrong. Maybe he was thinking of another baby when he wrote that?

Other parts of the discourse follow, "Feeding 55 CCs of formula every 4 hours. She is without feeding problems." Folks, I just have to stop here and say, "Thank you, Lord!" This is a complete reversal from last month!

Back to Dr. Cav: "Patient tends to get puffy at times - especially her feet and face. I would disregard this. No Lasix (diuretic) currently being given."

"Infant prone to be irritable and get apnea and brady. Was ventilator dependent during first month. Extubated herself on 7/4. Put on oxyhood. She is dependent on her oxyhood - a comforter of sorts! I've been trying to wean her to room air, but she resists. She needs to be forced to room air!"

Lastly, "Eyes need examining by Dr. D for possible RLF" (retrolental fibroplasia - a condition of the eyes that can happen in preemies who require excessively high levels of oxygen. The retina can convert into a fibrous mass.)

RLF was explained to me: lots of tiny blood vessels can develop in the eye when a baby is on oxygen-assisted ventilation. However, the blood vessels aren't very healthy. Over time, they can retract, shrivel, and die. This can pull the retina off the eye and cause blindness. So, Dr. D will be examining Janessa's eyes.

When August rolled in, it brought Dr. F into our lives. His handwriting is a little easier to decipher than Dr. Cav's. However, in Dr. F's lengthy "On Service Note," I noticed a major error. He said that Janessa hadn't had any bilirubin problem (jaundice) since birth. TOTALLY WRONG! The medical records clearly show that she has been under a "bili" light repeatedly for jaundice and increased bilirubin.

In fairness to Dr. F, though, I discovered why he wrote this. He got the incorrect information from Dr. Cav's "Off Service Note" that was written at the end of July. It said, "Bili - No problem since birth." So, even though Dr. Cav had noted Janessa's bilirubin problem when he first took over in July, he has now passed incorrect information to Dr. F.

To me, this incident clearly shows how easily wrong information can be dangerously passed down as fact. I believe this reveals the need for multiple medical personnel to put their eyes on these charts to help ensure that all previous notes are compared. Clearly, it is not enough to simply rely on the most recent posting. Janessa's bilirubin information might not have been an earth-shattering issue in this case. But, if it WERE something critical, an error like this could potentially cost someone their life.

August held quite a slate of developments, some minor and some major. On August 1, Janessa was placed upright in an infant seat for the very first time in her life. A nurse put the seat in Janessa's bed and sat her in it. According to the nurse, Janessa "tolerated it well, then became dusky. Her heart rate dropped into the 60s, and she required stimulation, then bagging." It's not clear how they gave Janessa oxygen while she sat in the infant seat. No notation. She was still requiring 25% oxygen under the oxyhood.

By August 2, Janessa weighed 4 1/2 pounds. An echocardiogram of her heart showed it to be perfectly normal! WHAT A GOOD REPORT!! The next day, her eyes were dilated and checked by Dr. D for any signs of RLF. It was determined that a recheck should be scheduled for two weeks, and he prescribed Vitamin E.

A case of diaper rash showed up in August, which caused the nurses to start using cloth diapers for Janessa. They surmised that she might possibly be sensitive to the plastic in disposable diapers. So, they discontinued using those, and the rash dissipated.

A monumental moment came on August 7. Janessa's oxyhood was removed, and she started breathing room air! After 69 days of oxygen assistance, she was now doing it all on her own!

While it had always been important to monitor Janessa's oxygen saturation, it continued to be critical at this point. The routine of drawing blood periodically to check her oxygen level continued after she was put on room air. However, her tendency to get irritated and fussy from the moment they first touched her caused her to get dusky, and this reaction adversely affected the lab results.

Here's the doctor's comments on the day after Janessa's switch to room air. "Blood gases aren't good. But child has good color at rest and doesn't seem to have any distress except when blood is drawn. Will leave on room air unless increased respiratory distress or poor color is noted."

Further notes read, "Baby fusses a lot when blood is drawn to check gases. Clinically does well with good color and no distress until feeding or lab work is drawn, then gets mildly cyanotic (blue). Will leave at room air, but give 25% oxygen with flow-by while feeding. Will quit following blood gases so often unless clinically indicated."

Even when another doctor filled in for the night, the same protocol was emphasized: "Blood gases on room air are sub-optimal (below acceptable level), but child was extremely agitated when blood was drawn. Will check skin oxygen monitor instead as a more benign (gentler) method of measuring oxygenation." So, it appears that Janessa's resistance to being stuck with needles is finally paying off!

She was moved to an isolette bed in another section of the perinatal center's huge room on August 10. Since she required less handling for tests and procedures, she no longer had to be kept in an open, radiant-warmed bed. An isolette has a clear, plastic, "hood" cover over the entire bed. There are round openings on the sides for nurses to reach through to tend the baby.

This bed was only home to Janessa for ten days. She was then graduated to a small, open crib due to her ability to maintain a constant body temperature without any assistance. At this time, her formula was changed to a brand that is commonly carried in most stores. This was done in preparation for her ultimate departure from the place where she had spent her entire little life.

There were a few problems, however, that lingered. During her feedings, it was still common for her to become dusky. So, a small tube of free-flowing oxygen was always held to her face while she took her bottle. There is a notation of this duskiness on August 20, just five days before her discharge from the hospital. Additionally, the very same problem is noted on August 25, THE DAY THEY SENT HER HOME! That notation reads,"Nippled only fair, with episode of duskiness during feeding."

Obviously, the nurse who fed her on this monumental day felt compelled to document Janessa's distress to make certain it is recorded that something is amiss.

Another unresolved problem is documented in the chart on August 22. Janessa had an episode where her heart rate dropping when she was feeding! While nurses in the perinatal center were excitedly talking about her soon release, shouldn't someone have been troubled at the thought of her leaving, given the ongoing symptoms that kept occurring?!

The doctor planned to do a 12-hour apnea test August 19. The test would take place while Janessa remained on theophylline (the medication that dilates air passages and stimulates cardiac and central nervous system activities). The test was conducted on that date. With the medication in Janessa's system, the test produced normal results.

A new test was then scheduled for a later date. It would be conducted WITHOUT the benefit of theophylline stimulating her system. Therefore, it would be necessary to stop the medication and allow sufficient time for the drug to leave her body before running the second test.

Something strange occurred on August 22, though, the day before the second test. I saw the following with my own eyes. A nurse prepared Janessa's feeding. She placed a dose of theophylline into the formula in the baby bottle and shook it. As she did, the formula turned a familiar light-brownish color, exactly as I had observed time and time again in the past.

This made no sense to me, since I had been told that the medication was stopped prior to this date to allow it to be completely out of Janessa's system for the new test. How could they possibly get an accurate reading of her ability to breathe on her own if this medication that stimulates breathing is still being given?

In hindsight, I realize that I should have brought this to someone's attention. But, at this time in my life, there was still a hesitation to question medical personnel. Plus, numerous things were happening rapidly in preparation for the dismissal, and I could hardly process everything.

For example, on August 23, Dr. D completed the recheck of Janessa's eyes. He ended up informing me that there appeared to be some very unhealthy progression of RLF. He would need to see her in his office right away after she came home. This was heartbreaking news to me.

To further add to my stress, a hearing test was conducted the very next day. For this procedure, a small, flat, metal bar that registers movement was placed under Janessa's thin mattress. Periodically, a "whoosh" sound would emanate from somewhere near the head of the bed. If she moved immediately after the sound occurred, the metal bar would record her movement, and the tech would document that Janessa heard the sound.

But, Janessa never moved at all when the noise sounded. Therefore, I was told that she scored so low on this test that it indicated she might be deaf!

Mind you, THIS earth-shattering news was thrown at me right after I'd gotten the bad news about Janessa's eyes. My entire world felt like it was unraveling at this point.

Now, back to August 23, the very next day after I had seen theophylline being put into Janessa's bottle. The second 12-hour apnea test was started at 11 AM.

Oddly, the report in the DOCTOR'S chart on the very next day (August 24) <u>WAS NOT WRITTEN BY A DOCTOR</u>; <u>IT WAS WRITTEN BY A NURSE</u>. It only says, "Recording normal - Monitor discontinued. Discharge in the morning." So, the day after this test, Janessa was removed from the heart and breathing monitor for the first time in her life.

Now, let me share some strange and concerning items from the ***DOCTOR'S*** *records AFTER the first test was done on August 19.*

There is a note for ***August 21*** *that says* ***theophylline was discontinued on August 20 (the day before)*** *in preparation for a second test.*

This note ***WAS NOT WRITTEN BY A DOCTOR. IT WAS WRITTEN AND SIGNED BY A NURSE... IN THE DOCTOR'S RECORD... ON AUGUST 21.***

But remember - I watched a nurse put theophylline in Janessa's bottle on AUGUST 22.

There is NO PAGE AT ALL in the DOCTOR'S RECORD for AUGUST 20 *(when the med was supposedly stopped).*

There IS a page for August 19 and one for August 21... ... but BOTH ARE WRITTEN BY THE SAME NURSE!

So, in a nutshell, a nurse is writing in the doctor's records saying that theophylline was stopped on August 20. No doctor wrote ANY notes in the doctor's records on these three days: August 19, 20, & 21. Notes that are written in the doctor's records for August 19 and 21 were written by ONE SPECIFIC NURSE. She wrote that the medication was discontinued on August 20, which is false.

The following is the last notation in Janessa's perinatal center nurse's chart. It is dated August 25, 1981, and it states, "Discharged home with mother. Accompanied and carried by NA to hospital entrance. Placed in car with mother. Baby in satisfactory condition." So, seven days before Janessa was even due to be born, she left the hospital after spending 87 days there.

Chapter 14

The Outcome

The little pink preemie dress that Janessa wore home absolutely swallowed her. She only weighed 5 pounds and 6 ounces. The fit of the dress didn't matter to me, though, because I was bringing my miracle home!

Her brother, Jeremy, had never been allowed into the perinatal center unit. He'd only had a few short glances at his baby sister through the famous glass window when I'd occasionally gotten to take him with me to the hospital.

There was a small isolated waiting room in which he had safely played while I went into the unit. During those few visits, Jeremy would sometimes briefly leave his playthings in that room and come softly knock on the window to wave at me. Now that Janessa was home, there was no glass separating Jeremy from his baby sister. What a wonderful feeling it was to finally have both of my children together.

At long last, I could breathe a sigh of relief. Or could I? Janessa had been given a clean bill of health by doctors in charge of her case. However, the uneasiness inside me kept urging me to check on her repeatedly when she was in her crib. A very slight "unction" kept nudging me. It wasn't fear. I just sensed that something wasn't quite right.

Well, four days after bringing Janessa home, the gentle leading would prove to be correct. On this day, I had fed her and was holding her as she slept. Suddenly, she completely stopped breathing and went limp in my arms.

Amazingly, I did not panic. Instead, I remembered the procedure I had watched the nurses perform again and again. I lifted one of Janessa's tiny little feet and repeatedly thumped the bottom of it with my thumb and finger over and over. Within a minute, she started to breathe, but it felt like an eternity. Relief rushed over me, but I knew this was very serious and very dangerous.

Immediately, I dialed the perinatal center phone number that was deeply embedded in my memory. I explained my emergency to the voice that answered. Shockingly, I was informed that Janessa could not be readmitted to the sterile environment of the perinatal center, since she had traveled into the outside world. She would instead need to be admitted to the regular pediatric floor of the hospital via a regular pediatrician.

WHAT?!! Janessa had never been to a pediatrician yet! She'd only been home for a few days. To the spokesperson's credit, she was very sympathetic and gave me the names and phone numbers of several pediatricians from which to choose. Of course, I could have used Jeremy's doctor, but I had grown dissatisfied with him and already decided to switch Jeremy's care elsewhere. This change of doctors was just being forced on me a little sooner than I'd anticipated.

After a quick phone call to the office of a pediatrician I chose from the list, I rushed Jeremy to my mom's house and headed to the hospital. From the many trips I'd made during the last three months, my car could have probably driven itself there by memory. In my wildest dreams, I never would have thought I'd be returning this soon. All the way there, I kept one hand on Janessa's chest to ensure I could feel her breathing.

Upon arrival at the hospital, I entered the Emergency Room and waited and waited. After the necessary protocol was completed in the ER, they finally admitted my tiny baby girl to the pediatric floor. In her room, she was immediately fitted around her tiny little chest with a foam belt that would monitor her breathing and her heart rate. Only then could I stop my own vigilant, manual observance of her breathing. Now, a machine would do that for me.

The new pediatrician decided that a repeat apnea test should be done. At this point, I informed him of my concern that theophylline had been given too close to the time of the last test. He assured me that this new test would be done correctly.

Lo and behold, when this test was conducted, apnea problems did indeed show up during the feeding portion. I expressed that these results now gave rise to a request that Janessa not leave the hospital this time without the safety net of a monitor. The doctor agreed. A few days later, I once again took my tiny baby girl home. This time, though, she was wrapped in a foam belt.

Within a week or so of bringing Janessa home again, it was time for Dr. D to recheck her eyes. So, we trekked to his office with the new portable monitor in tow. Sadly, this office visit did not bring good news. Due to the increased RLF symptoms in Janessa's eyes, Dr. D determined that it was absolutely necessary to re-hospitalize Janessa right away for a surgical procedure called cryosurgery. Time was of the essence, he explained, since RLF can progress very rapidly and totally destroy the retina.

He described cryosurgery as a process that involves putting tiny drops of liquid nitrogen around the outside edge of the retina. The liquid nitrogen literally freezes the spot it touches and "sears" and "seals" the retina to the eye ball. This ensures that the retina can never be pulled away from the eye by those tiny, unhealthy blood vessels that can shrivel and cause blindness.

So, on September 24, Janessa was readmitted to the hospital for surgery on her right eye. It was suggested that I just wait in her hospital room while she was taken for the operation. A short while later, I got a phone call from the doctor telling me that everything had gone very well with the procedure, and Janessa was being taken to the recovery room. He said she would be there about an hour and would then be returned to her room where I was waiting.

One hour passed, then two, then two and a half hours! By this time, I was growing VERY concerned and wanted to know where my baby was! For at least an hour, I had been regularly asking the nurse. Then, the phone rang in Janessa's room. When I answered it, I was shocked to hear the voice of Dr. B, one of the doctors from the perinatal center! He explained that he had been summoned to come quickly to the recovery room by Dr. D, because Janessa was unable to breathe on her own now!

When Dr. B arrived at the recovery room, he discovered they had used a breathing tube for Janessa during surgery that was far too small. She had gone through the entire surgery with an inadequate breathing tube, and now, she could not breathe on her own again!

Dr. B explained that this would be akin to only getting the amount of air that could flow through a straw when you need the amount of air that flows through a garden hose. Janessa had completely exhausted herself trying to get enough air during surgery and now needed a ventilator to breathe for her. Dr. B instructed them to intubate her with a larger breathing tube, which they had just done.

Because of the trauma to Janessa's system and the fact that she was now on a ventilator and could not breathe on her own, she was put into the INTENSIVE CARE UNIT! When they finally let me see her, I was horrified! She was heavily sedated and totally unconscious. Her eyes were black and blue, and she was hooked to a ventilator.

I must admit this was among the most traumatic things I had encountered since her birth. What was supposed to be a straightforward surgical procedure had turned into a nightmare for my tiny baby who couldn't breathe now and was in intensive care on a ventilator.

Amazingly, Janessa was able to successfully rebound from this catastrophic event and was released from the hospital two days later. My little five-pound baby girl was finally coming home again!

Janessa wore the apnea monitor belt for nine months. On at least three occasions, it proved to be a life saver for her. Each of those times, she stopped breathing entirely, and the monitor's warning alarm blared. I could respond quickly and get her breathing again. Words are inadequate to express how very grateful I was to have that monitor.

One doctor later speculated that Janessa might have been a "SIDS" baby even if she'd been born full term. He felt she was potentially one of the babies who would have stopped breathing in her bed. SIDS is Sudden Infant Death Syndrome and usually happens to a child under age one.

If I hadn't been watching her so carefully after bringing her home from the perinatal center, this story might have ended tragically. But, the reason I was on such high alert was due to her being born so prematurely and having such difficulties in the hospital. If she had not been premature, I doubt I would have felt the need to watch her so closely, and she might have died in her own crib.

Thankfully, we made it safely through the tedious nine months of monitoring, which required me to stay within sight or hearing distance of the alarm. I can remember putting the monitor on the window sill near her crib, so I could hang clothes on the clothesline outside and still see the flashing green lights.

Janessa came off the monitor around the time of her first birthday. However, it took me quite a while longer to fully relax and adjust to the fact that I no longer had the comforting assurance that her faithful monitor had provided.

For the first two or three years of her life, Janessa was taken periodically to the perinatal center's testing facility for evaluations of her physical and mental development. At first, we returned every three months or so, then every six months. To arrive at a fair standard by which to judge her development, they always deducted the three months of her prematurity from her actual age. That really didn't seem necessary, though, because she invariably scored far higher than her age, adjusted or not. Janessa absolutely amazed them every time.

As an adult now, she has no physical disabilities nor deficiencies at all. There are a few small marks on her body, though, as evidence of what she experienced. Both of her heels show where she had countless pricks for blood tests. There are a few tiny raised spots on her scalp where IVs were inserted, but her hair covers them. Lastly, there's the burn scar on her chest from the round oxygen sensor left too long in one spot in her first weeks of life.

These are the only physical traces of her prematurity that remain. Ironically, all of them are the result of medical treatment she received.

A picture of Janessa in adulthood is shown in this book as a living testimony to the goodness of God, and to the special gift of faith that was imparted to me for the duration of this entire situation. After the ordeal was over, that special manifestation of faith lifted, and I had to learn how to develop my own faith through the Word of God.

A "measure of faith" was given to me as a child, and I acted on that faith and became "born again" then. But, I had never let my faith develop. Well, all of that changed after I experienced God's amazing grace in the midst of this storm. I dived in to feed my faith and let it grow.

On Janessa's tenth birthday, I took her back to the perinatal center where we joined Heidi and her mother, Vicki. Remember Heidi? She's the other micro preemie who was born the very same night within minutes of Janessa and was exactly the same stage of prematurity. Both girls had been due on September 1. Yet, both were born on May 30. Another special link is the fact that Vicki and I had shared a hospital room together before our girls were born.

Let me tell you, when we showed up at the entrance of the perinatal center on the tenth birthday of these two miracles, the nurses and staff went wild! Several of the same nurses were still there and remembered vividly that dramatic night ten years earlier when two entire medical teams from the perinatal center were suddenly called to the delivery department within minutes of each other.

Of course, pictures were taken by a hospital photographer when we visited that day in 1991, and a story was soon published in the hospital newsletter. What a joy for these perinatal center "earth angels" (we'll call them) to see our daughters, who are living miracles.

Oh, by the way, remember that hearing test Janessa had failed in the perinatal center? Well, she was retested one month later at a specialist's office and passed with flying colors!

This doctor gave his professional opinion that the loud noises produced by alarms constantly sounding in the unit had more than likely conditioned Janessa to be so accustomed to a loud environment that she simply didn't respond at all to the gentle little "whooshing" sound made by the testing device. Yet, I had been given a terrifying report after the first test saying that my baby is likely deaf. Well, I'll say it again, "Thank you, God, that another negative report was totally turned around."

As a matter of fact, every negative medical report I ever received about her was completely turned around every time. Her health now can only be termed as "excellent!"

Looking back on the whole ordeal, I realize just how blessed I truly am that my daughter came through such traumatic and overwhelming circumstances with no lasting problems.

My ultimate response can be summed up like this:

"My baby was born too soon...

but not too soon for a miracle!"

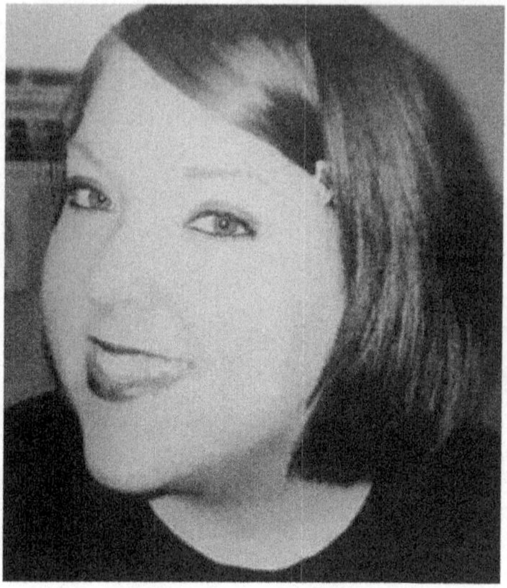

Janessa - Age 22

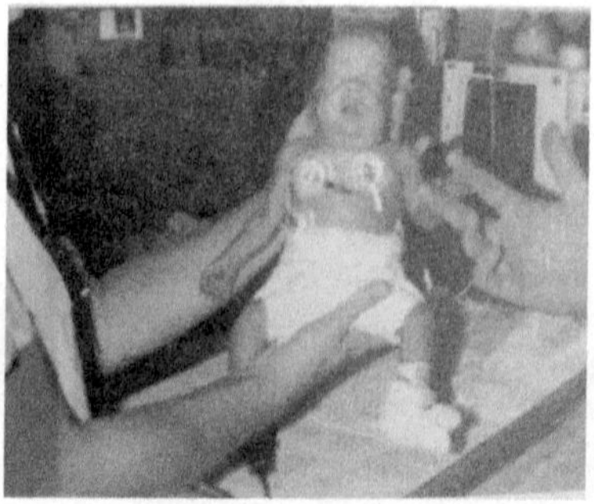

August 7
- 2 1/2 months old -

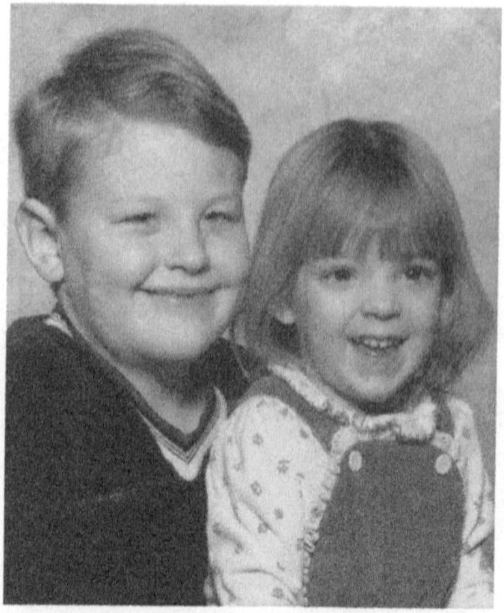

Jeremy - 6 Janessa - 2

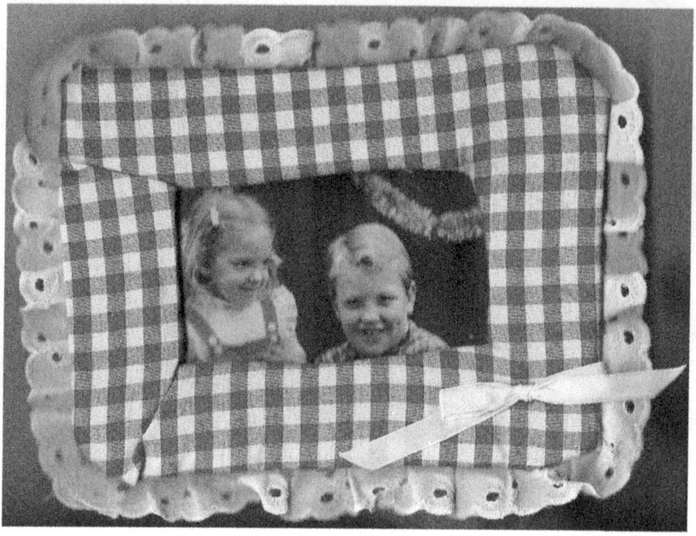

CHRISTMAS!
Jeremy - 7 Janessa - 3

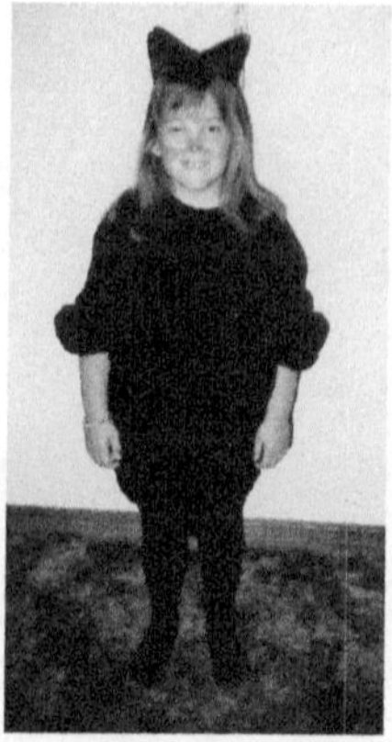

Piano Recital Song: Black Cat

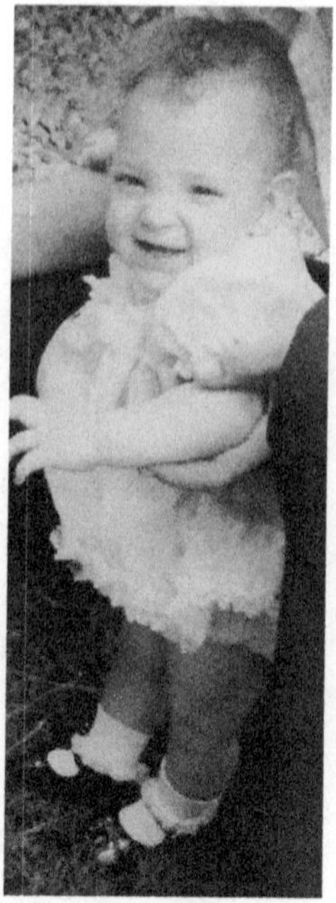

Age 1

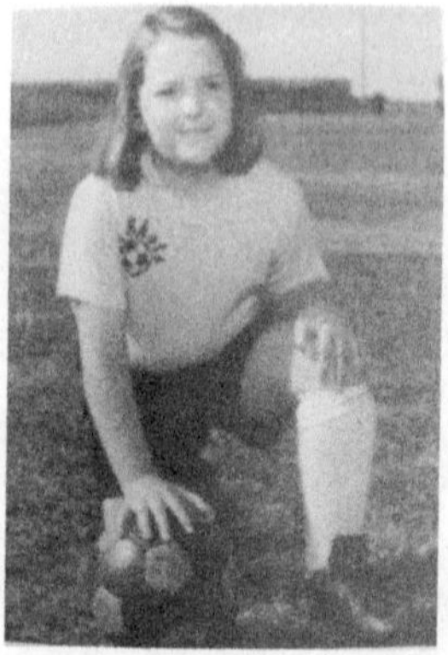

Soccer - age 9

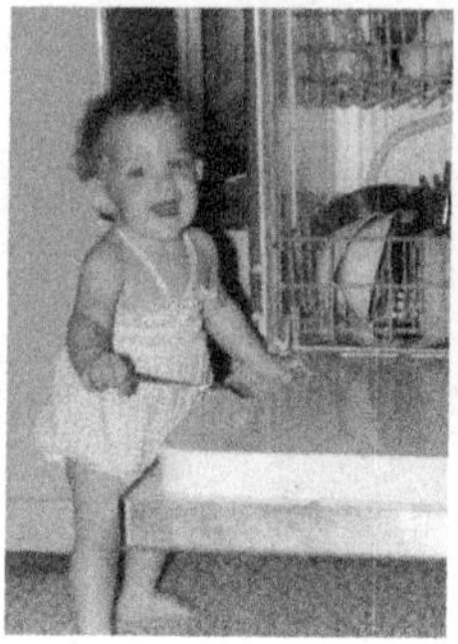

Age 1

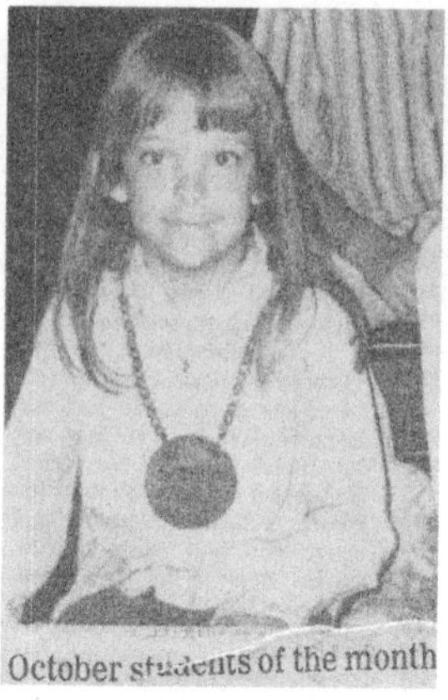

1st grade - Student of the Month

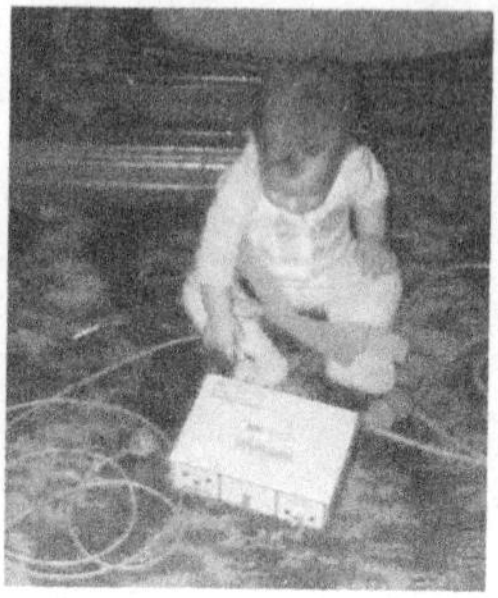

9 months old - inspecting monitor

PO Box 133 Owasso, OK 74055

Made in the USA
Monee, IL
04 November 2026

67377181R00069